The Mediterranean Diet Cookbook for Beginners

The Complete Mediterranean Diet Guide to Kick Start a Healthy Lifestyle

Includes:
Diet Rules and Guidelines
How to Start
14 Day Transition Menu Plan(Lose 10 lbs. in 14 Days)
90 Day (3 Month Menu Plan with Recipes)
100 Delicious and Easy Mediterranean Diet Recipes
Shopping List
Guidelines
What to Eat
What to Drink
Foods to Avoid

Susan Bradley M.D

Copyright© 2020
All Rights Reserved
ISBN: 9798588922623
Independently published

Disclaimer

While I draw on my prior professional expertise, background and personal experience in many areas, any recommendations I may make about weight training, nutrition, supplements or lifestyle in this book should be discussed between you and your doctor.
The information you receive in this guide do not take the place of professional medical advice.

Introduction

Every year, a team of panelists consisting of experts in nutrition, obesity, heart disease, and food psychology comes together to select the best and healthiest diet programs from amongst dozens of programs out there.

And for three years now, the Mediterranean diet has been named as the best diet program in the United States.

It was chosen as the best overall diet in 2018, 2019, and again in 2020.

The Mediterranean diet also ranked top in several other categories including:

Best Diets for Healthy Eating

Easiest Diets to Follow

Best Diets for Diabetes

Best Plant-based Diets

This is a big deal. Because, for any diet to be accepted by the medical industry, much less be voted as the best or healthiest diet, is no mean feat.

If you've ever had cause to discuss dieting with your doctor or nutritionist, you would agree with me that most of them typically frown at diet programs.

They would rather advise you to cut back on your calories, make healthier food choices, and exercise more, than have you go on a diet program, especially not one of those propagated on the internet as the next best thing.

Medical professionals typically frown upon yo-yo diets.

And with good reason too.

The truth is, most of these diet programs have dangerous side effects, especially when you do them over a long-term period.

You may end up doing your body more harm than good when you choose to embark on these diets.

Yes, you would lose weight but at what cost?

Most of these programs will have you cut off major classes of food that ought to supply your body with essential nutrients.

Carbohydrates are just as important to your body as proteins, fats, and every other class of food. So, when someone tells you not to eat carbs for 3 to 6 months so you can lose weight, they are pretty much telling you to deprive your body of some of the essential nutrients that it needs to thrive.

Yo-yo Diets will mess up your hormones, mess up your metabolism, tamper with your mood and mental health, and expose you to several potential health problems that often stem from nutrient deprivation.

For people who build their lifestyles based on yo-yo diets, health issues like osteoarthritis, digestive health problems, dementia, and skin disorders are usually not far behind, and that's why doctors hate them.

Let's not forget the fact that when you quit most of these diets and go back to eating normally again, you would often gain all of the weight back with a vengeance.

That's because your body system is not designed to run on 800 calories a day, or solely on proteins or fats.

It's just not going to work.

And numerous studies have revealed that 95% of people who embark on yo-yo diet programs are unable to sustain the results.

So, what's the point?

Why should you waste so much time and resources dieting- exposing their body to dangerous health risks, when the results aren't even sustainable?

No Doctor would want that for you, and that's why they typically warn you off diet programs.

Why the Mediterranean Diet Gets a Pass

Unlike most diet programs that are frowned upon in the health community, the Mediterranean diet is celebrated because it is not a diet program.

It is a healthy eating lifestyle that is sustainable over a long period.

The Mediterranean diet is based on the traditional eating pattern of a group of people who have been eating this way for thousands of years.

The people who traditionally eat this diet are typically healthy and free from many diseases, especially heart diseases that are common amongst people who eat the Standard American Diet, or other types of diets.

This was what led to the study and adoption of the Mediterranean diet as the best diet for weight loss, and heart health.

The Mediterranean diet is not a diet in the sense that it doesn't restrict you from eating any class of food or require any kind of calorie-counting.

All you need to do is eat like the Mediterranean people, and that's it- you get the results you are looking for, whether you're trying to lose weight, reverse aging, or improve your heart health.

In this book, we've laid out all the rules, tips, and guidelines that would help you get the best out of the Mediterranean diet as a beginner.

You'll learn:
- What The Mediterranean Diet is all About
- The Rules and Principles of the Mediterranean Diet
- The Health Benefits of the Mediterranean Diet
- How to Gradually Make The Switch from Your Present Diet to a Mediterranean Diet
- Foods to Eat on the Mediterranean Diet
- Foods to Avoid on the Mediterranean Diet
- How to Do the Diet If You're a Vegan, Vegetarian, or on a Plant-based Diet.
- Tips to Help You Create Your Own Personalized Menu Plan (Especially for People on a Budget)

You'll also find:

- A 14 Day Transition Menu Plan with Recipes to Lose Up to 10 lbs. in 14 Days.
- A 90 Day (3 Month) Mediterranean Diet Meal Plan with Recipes
- Shopping Lists and Where to Get Specialty Ingredients From.

How to Use This Guide

- **Understand the Diet:** The Mediterranean diet is not just a 2-week or 1-month challenge that you do once and abandon. It's a lifestyle.

    The idea is that you embrace this style of eating for the rest of your life so that you can live healthy without having to struggle with weight management every now and then.

    So, make sure you read the directions and understand them so that you can approach the diet the right way.

- **Understand The Benefits:** It helps to keep you motivated when you understand how the diet works, and what it's going to do to your body.

- **Learn How to Transition Gradually:** It's also important to introduce your body to this new lifestyle slowly and gradually.

    Remember, this is not a yo-yo diet so don't rush it.

    Use the tips in the guide to slowly switch from your current diet to a full Mediterranean lifestyle.

- **Use The 14 Day Menu Plan to Kick start The Diet and Lose 10 Pounds:** There's a specially crafted menu plan to help you kick start the diet when you're ready.

    The menu plan can also help you lose up to 10 pounds if you follow it religiously.

- **Use The 3 Month Diet Plan or Create Your Own Menu Plan Using the Recipes in The Book:** There's also a 3 month (90-day menu plan complete with breakfasts, lunch, dinner, and 2 snacks per day.

The menu plan will help you eat a Mediterranean diet for 3 months straight.

You can either follow this menu plan or create your own menu plan based on your budget.

There's a section that teaches you how to create your own menu plan according to your budget.

- **Use The Shopping List as a Guide:** There's also a comprehensive shopping list for both menu plans (the 14-day and 3-month plan) so you know what to buy when doing your grocery shopping.

Table of Contents

CHAPTER ONE — 13

WHAT IS THE MEDITERRANEAN DIET? — 13
HISTORY OF THE MEDITERRANEAN DIET — 13
HEALTH BENEFITS OF THE MEDITERRANEAN DIET — 17

CHAPTER TWO — 22

BASIC GUIDELINES OF THE MEDITERRANEAN DIET — 22
THE RULES AND PRINCIPLES OF THE MEDITERRANEAN DIET — 23
The Mediterranean Diet Food Pyramid — 23
HOW TO GRADUALLY MAKE THE SWITCH FROM YOUR PRESENT DIET TO A MEDITERRANEAN DIET — 27

CHAPTER THREE — 29

FOODS TO EAT ON THE MEDITERRANEAN DIET — 29

CHAPTER FOUR — 32

FOODS TO AVOID ON THE MEDITERRANEAN DIET — 32

CHAPTER FIVE — 34

14 DAY TRANSITION MENU PLAN WITH RECIPES TO LOSE UP TO 10 LBS. IN 14 DAYS — 34
SHOPPING LIST — 37

CHAPTER SIX — 39

HOW TO CREATE YOUR OWN MEDITERRANEAN DIET MENU PLAN (DIETING ON A BUDGET) — 39
TIPS FOR VEGANS AND VEGETARIANS — 40

CHAPTER SEVEN — 43

90 Day (3 Month) Mediterranean Diet Meal Plan — 43

CHAPTER EIGHT — 69

Mediterranean Diet Shopping List (and Where to Get Stuff From) — 69
Where to Get Mediterranean Diet Ingredients From — 72

BREAKFAST RECIPES — 74

- Blueberry Oats Bowl — 75
- Banana Yogurt Pots — 76
- Tomato and Watermelon Salad — 77
- Greek Burgers — 78
- Patsavouropita Cheese and Herb Pie — 79
- Sweet Potato and Feta Tart — 80
- Traditional Greek Feta Cheese Pie — 82
- Olive Phyllo Pies with Honey Syrup — 84
- Crispy Pita Bread with Feta Cheese Filling — 85
- Tahini-Feta Toast — 86
- Greek-Barley Rusks — 87
- Baked Olive Oil Croutons — 88
- Breakfast Shakshukka with Fresh Herbs — 89
- North African Breakfast Khlea and Egg — 90
- Isreali Breakfast Baba Ganoush — 91
- Israeli Breakfast Walnut Hummus — 92
- Israeli Overnight Breakfast Labane — 93
- Italian Breakfast Frittata — 94
- Italian Breakfast Couscous with Currants — 95
- North African Farka (Breakfast Pasta) — 96
- Semolina Pancakes with Honey Butter — 97
- Moroccan Breakfast Msemmen — 98
- Mediterranean Scrambled Eggs — 100
- Mediterranean Breakfast Quesadillas — 101
- Spicy Tuna Quesadilla — 102
- Mediterranean Breakfast Quinoa — 103

Low Carb Mediterranean Egg Muffins with Ham	104
Greek Goddess Bowl	105

LUNCH RECIPES — 106

Cannellini Bean Salad	107
Edgy Veggie Wraps	108
Carrot, Orange & Avocado Salad	109
Panzanella Salad	110
Quinoa & Stir-fried Veggies	111
Mixed Bean Salad	112
Moroccan Chickpea Soup	113
Mediterranean Hummus Pasta	114
Greek Kale Quinoa Chicken Salad	115
Pan Roasted Salmon	116
Tabbouleh Salad	117
Mediterranean Falafel Salad	118
Greek Rice Spanakokorizo with Spinach	119
Spetzofai Sausage and Peppers	120
Roasted Cauliflower with Cheese and Garlic	121
Greek Peas-Arakas Latheros	122
Tuscan Tomato and Bread Salad	123
Greek Marinated Anchovies	124
Pan-roasted Herbs and Garlic Crusted Sardines	125
Baked Phyllo Chips	126
Mediterranean Chicken Orzo	127
One Pan Healthy Paella	129
Greek Chicken Zucchini Noodles	131
Beef Stuffed Acorn Squash	132
Healthy Baked Ziti	134
Mediterranean Bento Bowl	135

DINNER RECIPES — 136

Moussaka	137
Spiced Tomato Baked Eggs	138
Salmon with Potato and Corn Salad	139
Spiced Carrot and Lentil Soup	140

Mediterranean Chicken Quinoa & Greek Salad	141
Grilled Vegetables with Bean Mash	142
Spicy Mediterranean Beet Salad	143
Honey Lemon Chicken Laps	144
Grilled Chicken Skewers served with Vegetable Salad	145
Cod and Asparagus Bake	146
Lemon Chicken with Asparagus	147
Sweet and Easy Herb- baked Sweet Potatoes	148
Cauliflower Rice with Rotini Pasta and Sausage	149
Classic Greek Lemon Roasted Chicken and Potatoes	150
Grilled Honey Harrissa Chicken Skewers served with Garlicky Mint Sauce	152
Greek-inspired Baked Mac and Cheese	153
Greek-styled Juicy Roasted Meatballs	154
Stewed Pork and Greens in Lemon Sauce	155
Greek Chicken Cooked in Diced Tomato	156
Roasted Veggies Pita Pizza	157
Italian Sheet Pan Eggs with Prosciutto and Artichokes	158
Israeli Yellow Chicken and Potatoes	159
Israeli Green Rice	160
Italian Hot Dish Dinner	161
Easy Pasta Skillet Dinner	162
Easy Minestrone Soup Dinner	163
Healthy Lasagna	164
North African Spiced Carrots	166
North African Spiced Shrimps with Couscous	167
One Pan Mediterranean Chicken	169
Smoky Tempeh Tostadas with Mango Cabbage Slaw	170
Sweet Potato Noodles with Almond Sauce	172
Conclusion	**174**

Chapter One

What is The Mediterranean Diet?

The Mediterranean diet is simply a Mediterranean-inspired approach to healthy living.

When you embark on the Mediterranean diet, you are simply mimicking the centuries-long dietary patterns of the Mediterranean people.

So, who are these Mediterranean people that we speak of?

The Mediterranean people are typically people who live in the over 20 countries that border the Mediterranean Sea.

Some of the Mediterranean countries include Italy, Spain, France, Israel, Greece, Albania, Algeria, Bosnia and Herzegovinian, Cyprus, Croatia, Lebanon, Malta, Libya, Turkey, Syria, Tunisia, Slovenia, Egypt, Montenegro, and Morocco.

However, the diet is based on the feeding patterns of only a few out of these countries.

A little history will help you understand better.

History of the Mediterranean Diet

It all began in 1948.

After the Second World War, there was so much poverty in Crete (Greece) that the Greek government had to invite a group of experts from the Rockefeller Foundation to conduct research on how to raise the standard of living.

The results of the research came as a surprise to the foreign researchers and the Cretans because the researchers found that the traditional diet of the Cretans was healthier and more nutritionally adequate than even the U.S standard diet.

The Cretan's traditional diet consisted majorly of fruits, beans, herbs, a lot of wild greens, wine, plenty of olive oil, and very little meat.

Enter Ancel Keys.

Ancel Benjamin Keys

Ancel Keys was an American Physiologist who dedicated his life to studying the impact of food on heart health.

For example, it was Ancel Keys who first discovered that saturated fat increases the risks of cardiovascular heart diseases.

During his numerous research efforts, Ancel Keys observed that the life expectancy of the Greek people was higher than any other country in the world.

According to the World Health Organization, the average life expectancy of a Greek was 45 years. Ancel Keys sought to know why.

Between 1958 and 1964 he embarked on a study now popularly known as the '7 Countries Study'.

The research was aimed at exposing the relationship between dietary patterns and the prevalence of coronary heart diseases.

During the study, he compared the dietary patterns in 7 countries including The United States, Japan, Italy, Greece, Finland, Netherlands, and the Former Republic of Yugoslavia which was made up of Bosnia and Herzegovina, Croatia, Macedonia, Montenegro, Serbia, the regions of Kosovo and Vojvodina, and Slovenia at the time.

During the study, he discovered some of the reasons why the Greek people had such high life expectancy rates. He found out that the good health that they enjoy was due to their diet.

Ancel Keys, along with his team of researchers, discovered that the countries around the Mediterranean had a unique type of diet that was associated with the low rates of coronary diseases, lower rates of cognitive decline, and low mortality rates obtainable amongst the people from the region.

After the study, Ancel Keys and his colleagues began promoting the diet of the Mediterranean people to Americans, and to his patients from all over the world who suffered from one coronary heart disease or the other.

The World Health Organization

In 1993, the World Health Organization began to show interest in the Mediterranean diet.

They teamed up with researchers from Harvard University and a non-profit organization called Oldways. The team of researchers was to conduct further research into the diet and figure out how to introduce the diet to the public.

It was this group of researchers that formally defined the diet, and created the Mediterranean Diet Food Pyramid that lists the guidelines of the diet including what foods to eat, and how to eat them to enjoy the health benefits of the diet.

The Mediterranean Diet Goes Viral

Around the year 2000, the Mediterranean diet grew in popularity and many Doctors and Health Practitioners around the world began prescribing the diet as a healthy and safe way to lose weight, protect heart health, stay healthy, and extend lifespan.

So, unlike most yo-yo diets that were 'formulated in the laboratory' by one health expert or researcher, this one wasn't created, it was discovered.

It is a way of life that has existed for thousands of years.

Scientists just saw a group of healthy people living a relatively long and disease-free life, checked out what they were doing, and began to encourage people to adopt a similar lifestyle.

This is why the Mediterranean diet is considered safe and healthy and continues to get awards and recommendations within the health community.

This is one diet that you can stay on for the rest of your life without worrying about risks or side effects.

Now let's talk about the health benefits of the Mediterranean diet- what does this diet do for your body?

Is it just a heart-friendly diet or can it help you lose weight?

How does it do that?

Let's start with weight loss because I know that's one thing a lot of people are interested in achieving.

Health Benefits of the Mediterranean Diet

1. Weight Loss and Weight Management

Because it focuses on the consumption of fresh, whole foods, the Mediterranean diet helps you lose weight safely and sustainably.

Many studies carried out on the subject have shown that the Mediterranean diet can help aid and speed up weight loss.

During a randomized clinical trial carried out in Israel, 322 moderately obese middle-aged participants, mostly men, were placed on three different diets.

One group was placed on a calorie-restricted low-carb diet, another group was on a calorie-restricted low-fat diet, and then a third group was placed on the Mediterranean diet.

While the average weight loss of participants placed on the low-fat diet was around 2.9kg, participants placed on the low-carb diet lost an average of 4.7 kg; those who did the Mediterranean diet lost 4.4kg on average.

People eating a Mediterranean diet lost more weight than people eating a low-fat diet, and people eating a Mediterranean diet lost a similar amount of weight as people eating a low-carb diet.

Don't forget that on the Mediterranean diet, there's no calorie counting or carb restriction, yet, the participants were able to lose almost as much weight as people who were on a restrictive diet.

2. Protects Against Type 2 Diabetes

The Mediterranean diet is very rich in fiber. When you consume a lot of fiber, your body absorbs food rather slowly and this, in turn, reduces blood glucose absorption and blood sugar spikes.

Your body can maintain a balanced sugar level, and this reduces the risks of type 2 diabetes.

Balanced blood sugar levels also reduce hunger and food cravings and that's another way that the Mediterranean diet helps to promote weight loss because the less food you eat (without starving yourself of course), the more weight you'll lose.

3. Prevents Cardiovascular Diseases and Stroke

There have been numerous studies on the subject and many of them have proven that the Mediterranean diet is indeed helpful for reducing the risks of heart diseases in humans.

One study was conducted over for five years and included 7,000 men and women in Spain who already had, or were at a high risk of developing cardiovascular diseases.

The participants of the study were required to eat a Mediterranean diet without calorie restriction throughout the study.

Their diets were particularly high in nuts and extra-virgin olive oil, and they were not required to perform any physical exercises for the study.

At the end of the study period, it was discovered that the participants had a 30 percent lower risk of developing heart diseases.

The participants who ate more extra-virgin olive oil and nuts had an even lower risk.

4. Protects Against Cancer

A review of 83 studies carried out on the subject was published in 2017.

The review was published in the Journal *Nutrients* in October 2017 and it showed that the Mediterranean diet is effective for reducing the risks of colorectal cancer and breast cancer, and can also help to reduce symptoms and mortality rates in patients already suffering from any type of cancer.

The researchers observed that these benefits were because the Mediterranean diet was rich in whole grains, vegetables, and a high fruit intake.

Another study published in the Journal of International Medicine in 2015 revealed that women who ate a Mediterranean diet supplemented with Extra-virgin olive oil had a 62 percent lower risk of suffering from breast cancer, compared to people who ate a low-fat diet.

5. Prevents Cognitive Decline and Alzheimer's Disease

Another scientifically proven health benefit of the Mediterranean diet is that it helps to reduce the decline in memory and reasoning skills that is typically associated with aging.

A scientific study sponsored by the National Institute on Aging, and published in May 2018, placed 70 people on the Mediterranean diet over 2 years.

At the end of the study period, the participants showed signs of improved cognition, reduced cognitive decline, and reduction in the onset of Alzheimer's disease.

6. Helpful for Patients with Rheumatoid Arthritis

Rheumatoid arthritis happens when the body's immune system erroneously perceives a threat and begins to attack the joints, causing swelling and pain around them.

The National Institute of Health's Office of Dietary Supplement recommends a diet rich in Omega 3 fatty acids found in fatty fish as one of the most effective ways to alleviate symptoms of Rheumatoid Arthritis.

The Mediterranean diet includes the consumption of several rich sources of Omega 3 fatty acids hence, is very helpful for patients suffering from Rheumatoid Arthritis.

7. Increases Longevity

The Mediterranean diet can also help to reduce risks of death and elongate lifespan by at least 20%.

People who live in regions where the Mediterranean Diet is traditionally eaten tend to have a higher lifespan but there are also scientific studies that prove that this isn't just a myth.

One research carried out by researchers from Harvard University included 4,000 women who consumed the Mediterranean diet rich in fruits, olive oil, nuts, vegetables, fruits, and fish, with minimally processed foods, red meats, and a moderate amount of wine and cheese, had a longer lifespan compared to a controlled group who were on the Standard American Diet.

8. Helps to Symptoms and Risks of Depression

The Mediterranean diet may also help combat symptoms of depression as confirmed by a study published in the Archives of General Psychiatry which involved 10, 094 Spanish adults.

The results of the study showed that subjects who closely followed the Mediterranean diet were more than 30% less likely to develop depression than those who least adhered to the diet.

The researchers explained that the individual components of the diet may improve blood vessel function, fight inflammation, reduce risks of heart diseases, and repair oxygen-related cell damaged, all of which may help reduce risks of developing depression or alleviate symptoms of depression in people already suffering from the mental health condition.

9. Slows Down The Process of Aging

The Mediterranean diet may also help slow down the process of aging due to the large presence of antioxidant foods in the diet.

Consuming a lot of natural antioxidants helps to prevent cell oxidation, which is the primary cause of aging in humans.

The body produces free radicals during normal metabolic processes but when there is an excess of these free radicals circulating in the body, it causes oxidative stress and leads to cell, protein, and DNA damage.

These damages are what typically cause accelerated aging in humans.

10. Combats Stomach Bloating and Helps to Give You a Flat Tummy

The Mediterranean diet also helps to improve gut health by improving gut flora.

This helps to combat Irritable Bowel Symptom (IBS), Gastrointestinal Diseases, Acid reflux, Gastric Dilatation Volvulus, and other conditions that cause stomach bloating.

11. Keeps You Agile

The Mediterranean diet also helps to reduce the risks of developing muscle weakness and other signs of frailty. It not only keeps you healthy but agile and strong too.

Chapter Two

Basic Guidelines of the Mediterranean Diet

Most of the rules and guidelines of the Mediterranean diet can be found in the Mediterranean diet food pyramid put together by Oldways (*remember Oldways? The research organization we talked about when we were discussing the history of the Mediterranean diet.*)

So, Oldways put this simple pictorial representation of the rules and guidelines of the Mediterranean diet together to help you understand the diet at a glance.

The Rules and Principles of the Mediterranean Diet

The Mediterranean Diet Food Pyramid

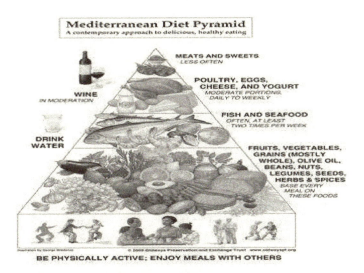

1. **Always Eat Breakfast**: Most people don't understand just how important breakfast is.

   Breakfast helps to activate your body's metabolism for the day.

   When you skip breakfast, it sends a signal to your body that there wouldn't be enough energy supply for the day and your body responds by slowing down your metabolism so that it can manage whatever it has to supply your body with much needed energy to function.

   But if you eat breakfast, it sends signal to your body that it's going to be a normal day (food and energy supply would come as usual) and so your metabolism is activated and continues to run as normal throughout the day.

On this diet, it is important to always have breakfast as skipping breakfast is often counterproductive.

2. **Daily Meals Should Be Based On Whole Grains, Fruits and Vegetables:** On the Mediterranean diet you don't need to count calories but you should ensure that most of your daily meals are built on the following:
   - Whole grains
   - Fruits
   - Vegetables
   - Beans
   - Nuts
   - Legumes
   - Seeds
   - Herbs and Spices

   You can eat as much of these as you want every day.

3. **Eat Fish and Seafood Twice a Week**: You should also aim to include healthy fish and seafood in your meals at least two times a week especially fish like tuna, salmon, herring, sablefish (black cod), and sardines which are rich in omega-3 fatty acids, and shellfish like mussels, oysters, and clams.

   You can have your fish anyhow you want; boiled, grilled, canned, air-fried but make sure you avoid deep-fried fish.

4. **Use Olive Oil as Your Major Source of Fat**: Instead of cooking with butter or other types of cooking oils, you should start cooking with olive oil instead.

   If you must cook with butter, use only unsalted butter and limit your consumption to no more than once a month.

5. **Limit Intake of Processed Foods**: Processed and packaged foods often contain a lot of chemicals that are used to preserve and package them so that they can hold up for long on the shelves.

These chemicals are often ingested during consumption and may end up as toxins in your body. Too many toxins in your body can cause cell damage, accelerated aging and may even cause cancer and several other health challenges.

Of course, it's almost impossible to not consume processed and packaged foods in today's world but you should limit your intake of them to the barest minimum.

It is also important to read the labels of whatever product you're buying so that you can be sure that they do not contain any notorious chemical additives.

6. **Consume Low to Moderate Amounts of Dairy Daily**: Dairy is fine, you can have dairy but in small quantities.

   A rule of thumb is to limit yourself to one or two dairy products in small quantities daily.

   So, you can't have milk and then cheese and then eggs and yogurt on the same day. Choose one or two items daily and have them in low to moderate quantities.

7. **Consume Low to Moderate Amounts of Eggs and Poultry Daily**: You can have eggs, chicken, and other poultry products daily on this diet but in low to moderate amounts.

8. **Eat Low Amounts of Red Meat Once a Month**: I know you love your steak but on the Mediterranean diet, you can't have red meat as often. You can only consume red meat once a month.

9. **Drink a Small Glass of Red Wine with Dinner Daily**: The Mediterranean people believe that red wine has a lot of health benefits so they consume a lot of it.

   Some recommend that you have a small glass with every meal but in order to avoid getting drunk during the day, I strictly advise that you only have it with your dinner.

10. **Drink At Least Eight 8-ounce Glasses of Water Daily**: Water is important too. To keep you hydrated, flush out toxins, and promote healthy metabolism.

    On the Mediterranean diet it is recommended that you have at least eight 8-ounce glasses of water every day. That's at least 2 liters of water daily.

11. **Eat Fruits for Dessert**: It's not that you can't have desserts on the Mediterranean diet but you can only have sweets and desserts once a month.

    So, you have to improvise by eating fruits for deserts. That's another smart way to get your daily quota of fruits in.

12. **Eat a Full Vegetarian Meal Once a Week**: Sometimes, help your body detoxify by eating a full vegetarian meal for a full day once a week.

    No meat, no fish, and no dairy products- just a good old veggie based meal.

13. **Be Physically Active**: The Mediterranean lifestyle is not limited to food intake alone. If you want to live a long and healthy life like the Mediterranean people, you have to be physically active too.

    Get at least 30 minutes of exercise daily. You can start with walking for only 30 minutes every day, and then gradually ramp it up until you've built a solid exercise routine for yourself.

14. **Enjoy Meals with Others**: The goal is to enjoy mealtimes. For the Mediterranean, meal times are not just about gulping down food but also times to unwind, de-stress, and spend quality time with friends and family.

How to Gradually Make the Switch from Your Present Diet to a Mediterranean Diet

Switching to a Mediterranean diet from your traditional diet is not always a walk in the park- You've spent most of your life eating a certain way and now you have to make a switch and it can be difficult.

That's why most people can't keep up with diet programs. They do it for a week or two and run back to their old way of eating.

You key is to not rush yourself when trying to switch to the Mediterranean diet. Take it slow and give yourself time.

You can even give yourself a month to transition. And during the transitioning period, start introducing yourself to the Mediterranean lifestyle little by little.

Here are a few things you can do to get yourself acquainted with the Mediterranean lifestyle:

- Start Sautéing your food in olive oil instead of butter and other oils.

- Start snacking on fruits and nuts.

- Include more fruits and vegetables in your diet by enjoying salad as a starter or side dish.

- Choose whole grains instead of refined breads, rice, and pasta.

- Substitute red meat for fish at least twice a week.

- Limit high-fat dairy by switching to skim or 1% milk from 2% or whole milk.

- Substitute chips, pretzels, crackers, and ranch dip with carrots, celery, broccoli and salsa.

- Substitute white rice with, quinoa and stir-fried meat with stir-fried vegetables and tofu.

- Substitute white bread sandwiches or rolls with sandwich fillings in whole-wheat tortillas.

- Substitute Ice cream with pudding made with skim or 1% milk.

Chapter Three

Foods to Eat on the Mediterranean Diet

The table below has a comprehensive list of foods that you should be eating on the Mediterranean diet.

The foods are divided into two categories:

- **Foods You Should Eat Liberally**: You can eat these foods everyday- as much as you want because they hold most of the nutritional benefits of the diet.

- **Foods You Should Eat in Moderation:** Although the Mediterranean diet is not a restrictive diet- you are pretty much allowed to eat anything you want but there are some foods that you are advised to eat in moderation.

  These foods are generally healthy but may contain some elements that when consumed in excess, may have negative effects on the body.

	Foods You Should Eat Liberally	Foods You Should Eat in Moderation
Grains	<ul><li>Oatmeal (Steel-cut or Old-fashioned)</li><li>Whole grain bread (made with whole wheat flour)</li><li>Quinoa</li><li>Bulgur Wheat</li><li>Farro</li></ul>	<ul><li>All bran cereal</li><li>Pasta</li><li>Polenta</li><li>Couscous</li><li>Whole grain crackers</li></ul>

Proteins	- Beans - Chickpeas - Tempeh - Lentils - Tofu - Seitan	- Eggs - Chicken - Seafood - Fish
Oils and Fats	- Extra-virgin olive oil - Olives - Avocado Oil - Avocado	- Canola Oil
Fruits and Veggies	- Zucchini - Dark Greens - Egg Plant - Artichokes - Bell Peppers - Blackberries - Peaches - Blueberries - Cherries - Raspberries - Apricots - Strawberries - Potatoes - Sweet potatoes - All root vegetables - Starchy Veggies	
Nuts and Seeds		- Almonds - Pistachios - Walnuts - Cashew Nuts - Pecans - Macadamia Nuts - Brazil Nuts - Hazel Nuts

			• Peanuts
Dairy			• Goat Cheese • Plain Greek Yogurt • Feta Cheese • Brie • Plain Ricotta • Milk • Cottage Cheese
Sweeteners			• Honey • Brown sugar (Small amounts of sugar added in coffee or tea)
Sauces and Condiments		• Pesto • Balsamic Vinegar • Tomato Sauce (sugar-free)	• Tzatzaki • Aioli • Tahini
Drinks		• Tea • Coffee • Water	• Red Wine • Alcohol
Herbs and Spices		• All dried herbs and spices • Garlic • All fresh herbs and spices	

Chapter Four

Foods to Avoid on the Mediterranean Diet

There isn't much to avoid on the Mediterranean diet. Like I've mentioned severally, this is not a diet that punishes you or deprives you of the foods you love.

It's okay to eat these items once in a while if you're craving them but it is best not to have any of the following items on your daily menu or eat them often:

Grains	Heavily processed grains including: • Pancakes • Frozen waffles • Crackers • Sugar sweetened cereals
Proteins	• Bacon • Red meat (such as pork or beef) • Processed meat or meat products (e.g. chicken nuggets)
Oils and Fats	• Butter • Trans fat • Margarine
Nuts and Seeds	• Sugar-coated nuts • Sweetened mixed nuts • Sweetened nut butter

Dairy	- Ice cream
- Processed cheese (e.g. American)
- Sweetened Yogurt
Sweeteners	- White sugar
Sauces and Condiments	- Ketchup
- Barbecue sauce
- Teriyaki sauce
Drinks	- Fruit juice
- Soda
- Bottled or canned sweetened coffee

Chapter Five

14 Day Transition Menu Plan with Recipes to Lose Up To 10 Lbs. in 14 Days

	Week 1				
	Breakfast	Lunch	Snack	Dinner	Late Night Snack
Day 1	Blueberry Oats Bowl	Cannellini Bean Salad	One handful of Preferred Nuts	Moussaka	One Cup of Preferred Fruits
	2 Cups of Water	2 Cups of Water	2 cups of water	1 cup of water	1 cup of water
				1 small glass of red wine	
Day 2	Banana Yogurt Pots	Cannellini Bean Salad	One handful of Preferred Nuts	Moussaka	One Cup of Preferred Fruits
	2 Cups of Water	2 Cups of Water	2 Cups of Water	1 cup of water	1 cup of water
				1 small glass of red wine	
Day 3	Tomato and Watermelon Salad	Edgy Veggie Wraps	One handful of Preferred Nuts	Spiced Tomato Baked Eggs	One Cup of Preferred Fruits
	2 Cups of Water	2 Cups of Water	2 Cups of Water	1 cup of water	1 cup of water
				1 small glass of red wine	
Day 4	Banana Yogurt Pots	Edgy Veggie Wraps	One handful of Preferred Nuts	Spiced Tomato Baked Eggs	One Cup of Preferred Fruits
	2 Cups of Water	2 Cups of Water	2 Cups of Water	1 cup of water	1 cup of water
				1 small glass of red wine	
Day 5	Tomato and	Carrot,	One	Salmon	One Cup

	Watermelon Salad	Orange & Avocado Salad	handful of Preferred Nuts	with Potato and Corn Salad	of Preferred Fruits
	2 Cups of Water	2 Cups of Water	2 Cups of Water	1 cup of water	1 cup of water
				1 small glass of red wine	
Day 6	Blueberry Oats Bowl	Carrot, Orange & Avocado Salad	One handful of Preferred Nuts	Spiced Carrot and Lentil Soup	One Cup of Preferred Fruits
	2 Cups of Water	2 Cups of Water	2 Cups of Water	1 cup of water	1 cup of water
				1 small glass of red wine	
Day 7	Greek Burgers	Panzanella Salad	One handful of Preferred Nuts	Spiced Carrot and Lentil Soup	One Cup of Preferred Fruits
	2 Cups of Water	2 Cups of Water	2 Cups of Water	1 cup of water	1 cup of water
				1 small glass of red wine	

	Week 2				
	Breakfast	Lunch	Snack	Dinner	Late Night Snack
Day 1	Sweet Potato and Feta Tart	Panzanella Salad	One handful of Preferred Nuts	Mediterranean Chicken Quinoa & Greek Salad	One Cup of Preferred Fruits
	2 Cups of Water	2 Cups of Water	2 cups of water	1 cup of water	1 cup of water
				1 small glass of red wine	
Day 2	Greek Burgers	Quinoa & Stir-fried Veggies	One handful of Preferred Nuts	Mediterranean Chicken Quinoa & Greek Salad	One Cup of Preferred Fruits
	2 Cups of Water	2 Cups of Water	2 cups of water	1 cup of water	1 cup of water
				1 small glass of red wine	
Day 3	Crispy Pita Bread with Feta Cheese Filling	Quinoa & Stir-fried Veggies	One handful of Preferred Nuts	Grilled Vegetables with Bean Mash	One Cup of Preferred Fruits
	2 Cups of	2 Cups of	2 cups of	1 cup of water	1 cup of

	Water	Water	water		water
				1 small glass of red wine	
Day 4	Italian Breakfast Frittata	Mixed Bean Salad	One handful of Preferred Nuts	Grilled Vegetables with Bean Mash	One Cup of Preferred Fruits
	2 Cups of Water	2 Cups of Water	2 cups of water	1 cup of water	1 cup of water
				1 small glass of red wine	
Day 5	Crispy Pita Bread with Feta Cheese Filling	Mixed Bean Salad	One handful of Preferred Nuts	Salmon with Potato and Corn Salad	One Cup of Preferred Fruits
	2 Cups of Water	2 Cups of Water	2 cups of water	1 cup of water	1 cup of water
				1 small glass of red wine	
Day 6	Italian Breakfast Frittata	Moroccan Chickpea Soup	One handful of Preferred Nuts	Spicy Mediterranean Beet Salad	One Cup of Preferred Fruits
	2 Cups of Water	2 Cups of Water	2 cups of water	1 cup of water	1 cup of water
				1 small glass of red wine	
Day 7	Sweet Potato and Feta Tart	Moroccan Chickpea Soup	One handful of Preferred Nuts	Spicy Mediterranean Beet Salad	One Cup of Preferred Fruits
	2 Cups of Water	2 Cups of Water	2 cups of water	1 cup of water	1 cup of water
				1 small glass of red wine	

Shopping List

(For 2 Servings of each meal)

Dairy	Qty	Bakery	Qty
Eggs	4	Wholemeal Loaf of Bread	1
Milk	60 ml / ¼ cup	Wholemeal Tortillas	2
Feta Cheese	350 g / 2 ⅓ cups		
Greek Yogurt	1300 g / 4 ⅓ cups		

Meat & Fish		Spices & Herbs	
Salmon Fillets	2	Crushed Red Chilli Flakes	Ground Cumin
Lean Beef Mince	250 g / 9 oz	Cumin Seed	Ground Cinnamon
Chicken Breasts	2	Fresh Coriander / Cilantro	Fresh Basil —
		Fresh Parsley —	Fresh Mint
		Tumeric	Rocket / Arugula —
		Sumac	

Condiments and Pantry Supplies		Fruits, Nuts, & Veggies	
Vegetable Stock	1000 ml / 4 ¼ cup	Walnuts	45 g / 6 tbsp
Tomato Puree — —		Split Red Lentils	70 g / ⅓ cup
Cannellini Beans	800 g / 4 cups	Aubergine / Eggplant	1
Sundried Tomato Paste		Black Olives	50 g / ¼ cup —
Capers	—8 g / 1 tbsp	Avocados	2 —
Red Wine Vinegar —		Baby Beetroot	8
Canned Tomatoes	1200 g / 6 cups	Artichoke Hearts —	145 g / ⅘ cup
Quinoa	200 g / 1 ⅙ cups	Bananas	6
Chickpeas	800 g / 4 cups —	Zucchini / Courgette	
Porridge Oats	120 g / 1 ⅓ cups —	Bell Pepper	1
Extra Virgin Olive Oil		Watermelon	1
Hummus —		Broad Beans	50 g / ¼ cups
Honey		Broccoli Head	1
Harrisa Paste		Sweetcorn Cob	1
Haricot Beans	400 g / 2 cups	Blueberries	350 g / 3 ½ cups
		Spring Onions / Scallions	

Carrots	500 g / 4 ½ cups
Red Chillis	2
Celery Stick	1
Oranges	2
Onions	5 —
New Potatoes	200 g / 1 ⅓ cups
Cherry Tomatoes	1220 g / 6 ⅛ cups
Lemons	2
Cucumber	1
Leek	150 g / 1 ⅔ cups —
Garlic Clove	1 —

Chapter Six

How to Create Your Own Mediterranean Diet Menu Plan (Dieting on a Budget)

Healthy eating is often more expensive than regular eating. When you choose to start eating healthy, your choices become limited. You can't just walk into a fast-food and get a $10 meal. You have to start cooking most of your meals and that means that you would have to buy a whole lot of ingredients and condiments.

It's even pricier when you have to follow a pre-designed menu plan.

But don't worry- if you can't afford to follow a pre-designed menu plan, you can come up with your own plan using the guide below.

Choose and plan your meals according to what you can afford.

Breakfast	<ul><li>Choose a Whole-grain based breakfast</li><li>Add one dairy product(e.g. milk or cheese)</li><li>Add one poultry product(e.g. eggs or chicken)</li><li>2 Glasses of Water</li></ul>
Mid-day Snack	<ul><li>Choose a handful of your preferred nuts</li><li>1 Glass of Water</li></ul>
Lunch	<ul><li>Choose a Veggie based meal for</li></ul>

	lunch (e.g. salad or veggie soup). • 2 Glasses of Water
Evening Snack	• 1 Cup of Your Preferred fruit • 1 Glass of Water
Dinner	• Choose a Beans or legume based dinner • Add a lot of herbs to your dinner • 2 Glasses of water • 1 small glass of red wine
Late Night Snack	• A small bowl or fruit salad (You can have this as dessert with your dinner instead). • One Small serving of unsweetened Greek yogurt • 1 glass of water

- Choose the days when you would have fish and seafood (remember you need to include these in your diet twice a week).

- Choose the days when you would your small serving of red meat once a month.

- Choose when and what sweets to have once a month e.g. sugar, honey, maple syrup.

Tips for Vegans and Vegetarians

One of the things I love about the Mediterranean diet is that vegans and vegetarians can easily do it too because the diet naturally limits the consumption of meat, and focuses on legumes, vegetables, and whole grains.

As a vegan, chances are pretty good that you already eat many of the foods considered part of the Mediterranean diet.

Here are a few tips that would help you enjoy the Mediterranean even on a plant-based diet.

- **Eat a Lot of Beans for Protein**: Beans are a great way to get protein, fiber, and prevent heart disease, according to the American Heart Association. They are also a vital component of the Mediterranean diet.

    To get your legume fix, try mixing some beans (like chickpeas, black beans, kidney beans, lentils, or peas) in a salad, soup, or platter of sautéed veggies. Just make sure you do rinse them because this helps to minimize sodium.

- **Nuts and Seeds are a Good Substitute for Fish and Seafood**: The Diet recommends that you eat fish and seafood at least twice a week to supply Omega-3 fatty acids.

    As someone on a plant-based diet, you can get your omega-3 from nuts and seeds like hemp seeds, chia seeds, walnuts, and flax seeds.

- **Substitute Tofu for Meat**: Of course, you need a lot of protein on this diet but tofu is just as good as any source of animal protein.

    You can get enough protein by adding small portions of tofu (made of soya beans) to your meals few times a week.

- **Whole Grains Add More Fiber to Your Diet**: Choose whole grain sources like sprouted bread, whole-wheat pasta, bread, and quinoa as they add fiber to your diet and help you stay fuller and more satisfied for a longer period of time.

- **Satisfy Your Sweet Tooth with Fruit**: Sugar cravings are normal but since the Mediterranean diet limits the consumption of sugar, you can get your sweet fix from fruits that have a lot of natural sugar such as oranges, grapefruit, raspberries, and blackberries.

These fruits also contain a lot of vitamins and antioxidants that are very beneficial for your body.

Here's a comprehensive list of plant-based food substitutes you can try:

Whole grains: Quinoa, brown rice, old-fashioned rolled oats, whole-wheat pita bread, whole-grain bread.

Plant-based protein: Black beans, chickpeas, hummus, lentils, tofu.

Nuts & seeds: Pecans, almonds, cashews, chia seeds, tahini.

Other healthy fats: Avocado, olives, olive oil.

Fruit: Apples, pears, clementines, dried figs, dried apricots, tomatoes.

Vegetables: Edamame, kale, Brussels sprouts, cabbage, cucumbers, peppers, garlic, ginger, onion, artichoke hearts, salad greens, carrots, spinach, broccoli, mushrooms, shallots, zucchini, sweet potatoes, corn.

Fresh herbs: Cilantro, parsley, oregano, chives.

Spices: Turmeric, cumin, chipotle powder.

Dairy alternatives: Unsweetened soy, almond and coconut milks.

Chapter Seven

90 Day (3 Month) Mediterranean Diet Meal Plan

MONTH ONE

Week One

	Breakfast	Lunch	Snack	Dinner	Late Night Snack (or dessert)
Quantity	One Serving	One Serving	One Handful	One Serving	As much as you can eat or make into smoothie
Day 1	Greek Burgers	Mediterranean Hummus Pasta	Black Sesame seeds	Honey Lemon Chicken Laps 1 small glass of red wine	Avocado
	2 glasses of water	2 glasses of water	2 glasses of water	1 small glass of red wine 1 glass of water	1 glass of water

Day 2	Patsavouropita Cheese and Herb Pie	Greek Kale Quinoa Chicken Salad	Pine nuts	Grilled Chicken Skewers served with Vegetable Salad	Oranges	
	2 glasses of water	2 glasses of water	2 glasses of water	1 small glass of red wine	1 glass of water	
				1 glass of water		
Day 3	Sweet Potato and Feta Tart	Pan Roasted Salmon	Walnuts	Cod and Asparagus Bake	Apples	
	2 glasses of water	2 glasses of water	2 glasses of water	1 small glass of red wine	1 glass of water	
				1 glass of water		
Day 4	Traditional Greek Feta Cheese Pie	Tabbouleh Salad	Black Sesame seeds	Lemon Chicken with Asparagus	Watermelon	
				1 small glass of red wine	1 glass of water	
			2 glasses of water	1 glass of water		
	2 glasses of water	2 glasses of water	2 glasses of water	1 small glass of red wine	1 glass of water	
				1 glass of		

				water	
Day 5	Olive Phyllo Pies with Honey Syrup	Mediterranean Falafel Salad	Pine nuts	Sweet and Easy Herb-baked Sweet Potatoes	Strawberries
	2 glasses of water	2 glasses of water	2 glasses of water	1 small glass of red wine	1 glass of water
				1 glass of water	
Day 6	Crispy Pita Bread with Feta Cheese Filling	Greek Rice Spanakokorizo with Spinach	Walnuts	Cauliflower Rice with Rotini Pasta and Sausage	Blueberries
	2 glasses of water	2 glasses of water	2 glasses of water	1 small glass of red wine	1 glass of water
				1 glass of water	
Day 7	Tahini-Feta Toast	Spetzofai Sausage and Peppers	Black Sesame seeds	Classic Greek Lemon Roasted Chicken and Potatoes	Apples
	2 glasses of water	2 glasses of water	2 glasses of water	1 small glass of red wine	1 glass of water
				1 glass of	

water

		Week Two			
	Breakfast	Lunch	Snack	Dinner	Late Night Snack (or dessert)
Quantity	One Serving	One Serving	One Handful	One Serving	As much as you can eat or make into smoothie
Day 1	Greek-Barley Rusks	Roasted Cauliflower with Cheese and Garlic	Pistachios	Grilled Honey Harrissa Chicken Skewers served with Garlicky Mint Sauce	Avocado
	2 glasses of water	2 glasses of water	2 glasses of water	1 small glass of red wine 1 glass of water	1 glass of water
Day 2	Baked Olive Oil Croutons	Greek Peas-Arakas Latheros	Hazelnuts	Greek-inspired Baked Mac and Cheese	Oranges
	2 glasses of water	2 glasses of water	2 glasses of water	1 small glass of red wine 1 glass of water	1 glass of water
Day 3	Breakfast Shakshukka with Fresh Herbs	Tuscan Tomato and Bread Salad	Almonds	Greek-styled Juicy Roasted Meatballs	Apples
	2 glasses of water	2 glasses of water	2 glasses of water	1 small glass of red wine 1 glass of water	1 glass of water
Day 4	North African Breakfast Khlea and Egg	Greek Marinated Anchovies	Pistachios	Stewed Pork and Greens in Lemon Sauce	Watermelon
	2 glasses of water	2 glasses of water	2 glasses of water	1 small glass of red wine 1 glass of water	1 glass of water

Day 5	Isreali Breakfast Baba Ganoush	Pan-roasted Herbs and Garlic Crusted Sardines	Hazelnuts	Greek Chicken Cooked in Diced Tomato of water	Strawberries
	2 glasses of water	2 glasses of water	2 glasses of water	1 small glass of red wine 1 glass of water	1 glass of water
Day 6	Israeli Breakfast Walnut Hummus	Baked Phyllo Chips	Almonds	Roasted Veggies Pita Pizza	Blueberries
	2 glasses of water	2 glasses of water	2 glasses of water	1 small glass of red wine 1 glass of water	1 glass of water
Day 7	Israeli Overnight Breakfast Labane	Mediterranean Chicken Orzo	Pistachios	Italian Sheet Pan Eggs with Prosciutto and Artichokes	Apples
	2 glasses of water	2 glasses of water	2 glasses of water	1 small glass of red wine 1 glass of water	1 glass of water

	Week Three				
	Breakfast	Lunch	Snack	Dinner	Late Night Snack (or dessert)
Quantity	One Serving	One Serving	One Handful	One Serving	As much as you can eat or make into smoothie
Day 1	Italian Breakfast Frittata	One Pan Healthy Paella	Pecans	Israeli Yellow Chicken and Potatoes	Avocado
	2 glasses of water	2 glasses of water	2 glasses of water	1 small glass of red wine 1 glass of water	1 glass of water
Day 2	Italian Breakfast Couscous with Currants	Greek Chicken Zucchini Noodles	Dates	Israeli Green Rice	Oranges
	2 glasses of water	2 glasses of water	2 glasses of water	1 small glass of red wine 1 glass of water	1 glass of water
Day 3	North African Farka (Breakfast Pasta)	Beef Stuffed Acorn Squash	Peanuts	Italian Hot Dish Dinner	Apples
	2 glasses of water	2 glasses of water	2 glasses of water	1 small glass of red wine 1 glass of water	1 glass of water
Day 4	Semolina Pancakes with Honey Butter	Healthy Baked Ziti	Pecans	Easy Pasta Skillet Dinner	Watermelon
	2 glasses of water	2 glasses of water	2 glasses of water	1 small glass of red wine 1 glass of water	1 glass of water
Day 5	Morrocan Breakfast Msemmen	Mediterranean Bento Bowl	Dates	Easy Minestrone Soup Dinner	Strawberries
	2 glasses of water	2 glasses of water	2 glasses of water	1 small glass of red wine 1 glass of water	1 glass of water
Day 6	Mediterranean Scrambled Eggs	Cannellini Bean Salad	Peanuts	Healthy Lasagna	Blueberries

Day 7	2 glasses of water	2 glasses of water	2 glasses of water	1 small glass of red wine 1 glass of water	1 glass of water
	Mediterranean Breakfast Quesadillas	Edgy Veggie Wraps	Pecans	North African Spiced Carrots	Apples
	2 glasses of water	2 glasses of water	2 glasses of water	1 small glass of red wine 1 glass of water	1 glass of water

	Week Four				
	Breakfast	Lunch	Snack	Dinner	Late Night Snack (or dessert)
Quantity	One Serving	One Serving	One Handful	One Serving	As much as you can eat or make into smoothie
Day 1	Spicy Tuna Quesadilla	Carrot, Orange & Avocado Salad	Cashew Nuts 2 glasses of water	North African Spiced Shrimps with Couscous	Avocado
	2 glasses of water	2 glasses of water	2 glasses of water	1 small glass of red wine 1 glass of water	1 glass of water
Day 2	Mediterranean Breakfast Quinoa	Panzanella Salad	Macadamia Nuts	One Pan Mediterranean Chicken	Oranges
	2 glasses of water	2 glasses of water	2 glasses of water	1 small glass of red wine 1 glass of water	1 glass of water
Day 3	Low Carb Mediterranean Egg Muffins with Ham	Quinoa & Stir-fried Veggies	Brazil Nuts	Smoky Tempeh Tostadas with Mango Cabbage Slaw	Apples
	2 glasses of water	2 glasses of water	2 glasses of water	1 small glass of red wine 1 glass of water	1 glass of water
Day 4	Greek Goddess Bowl	Mixed Bean Salad	Peanuts	Sweet Potato Noodles with Almond Sauce	Watermelon
	2 glasses of water	2 glasses of water	2 glasses of water	1 small glass of red wine 1 glass of water	1 glass of water
Day 5	Blueberry Oats Bowl	Moroccan Chickpea Soup	Cashew Nuts	Spicy Mediterranean Beet Salad	Strawberries
	2 glasses of water	2 glasses of water	2 glasses of water	1 small glass of red wine 1 glass of water	1 glass of water
Day 6	Banana Yogurt Pots	Cannellini Bean Salad	Macadamia Nuts	Moussaka	Blueberries
	2 glasses of water	2 glasses of water	2 glasses of water	1 small glass of red wine 1 glass of water	1 glass of water
Day 7	Tomato and Watermelon Salad	Edgy Veggie Wraps	Brazil Nuts	Spiced Tomato Baked Eggs	Apples

| | 2 glasses of water | 2 glasses of water | 2 glasses of water | 1 small glass of red wine
1 glass of water | 1 glass of water |

MONTH TWO

Week Five

	Breakfast	Lunch	Snack	Dinner	Late Night Snack (or dessert)
Quantity	One Serving	One Serving	One Handful	One Serving	As much as you can eat or make into smoothie
Day 1	Greek-Barley Rusks	Roasted Cauliflower with Cheese and Garlic	Black Sesame seeds	Grilled Honey Harrissa Chicken Skewers served with Garlicky Mint Sauce	Avocado
	2 glasses of water	2 glasses of water	2 glasses of water	1 small glass of red wine 1 glass of water	1 glass of water
Day 2	Baked Olive Oil Croutons	Greek Peas-Arakas Latheros	Pine nuts	Greek-inspired Baked Mac and Cheese	Oranges
	2 glasses of water	2 glasses of water	2 glasses of water	1 small glass of red wine 1 glass of water	1 glass of water
Day 3	Breakfast Shakshukka with Fresh Herbs	Tuscan Tomato and Bread Salad	Walnuts	Greek-styled Juicy Roasted Meatballs	Apples
	2 glasses of water	2 glasses of water	2 glasses of water	1 small glass of red wine 1 glass of water	1 glass of water
Day 4	North African Breakfast Khlea and Egg	Greek Marinated Anchovies	Black Sesame seeds	Stewed Pork and Greens in Lemon Sauce	Watermelon
	2 glasses of water	2 glasses of water	2 glasses of water	1 small glass of red wine 1 glass of water	1 glass of water
Day 5	Isreali Breakfast Baba	Pan-roasted Herbs and Garlic Crusted	Pine nuts	Greek Chicken Cooked in	Strawberries

	Ganoush	Sardines		Diced Tomato	
	2 glasses of water	2 glasses of water	2 glasses of water	1 small glass of red wine 1 glass of water	1 glass of water
Day 6	Israeli Breakfast Walnut Hummus	Baked Phyllo Chips	Walnuts	Roasted Veggies Pita Pizza	Blueberries
	2 glasses of water	2 glasses of water	2 glasses of water	1 small glass of red wine 1 glass of water	1 glass of water
Day 7	Israeli Overnight Breakfast Labane	Mediterranean Chicken Orzo	Black Sesame seeds	Italian Sheet Pan Eggs with Prosciutto and Artichokes	Apples
	2 glasses of water	2 glasses of water	2 glasses of water	1 small glass of red wine 1 glass of water	1 glass of water

	Week Six				
	Breakfast	Lunch	Snack	Dinner	Late Night Snack (or dessert)
Quantity	One Serving	One Serving	One Handful	One Serving	As much as you can eat or make into smoothie
Day 1	Greek Burgers	Mediterranean Hummus Pasta	Pistachios	Honey Lemon Chicken Laps	Avocado
	2 glasses of water	2 glasses of water	2 glasses of water	1 small glass of red wine 1 glass of water	1 glass of water
Day 2	Patsavouropita Cheese and Herb Pie	Greek Kale Quinoa Chicken Salad	Hazelnuts	Grilled Chicken Skewers served with Vegetable Salad	Oranges
	2 glasses of water	2 glasses of water	2 glasses of water	1 small glass of red wine 1 glass of water	1 glass of water
Day 3	Sweet Potato and Feta Tart	Pan Roasted Salmon	Almonds	Cod and Asparagus Bake	Apples
	2 glasses of water	2 glasses of water	2 glasses of water	1 small glass of red wine 1 glass of water	1 glass of water
Day 4	Traditional Greek Feta Cheese Pie	Tabbouleh Salad	Pistachios	Lemon Chicken with Asparagus	Watermelon
	2 glasses of water	2 glasses of water	2 glasses of water	1 small glass of red wine 1 glass of water	1 glass of water
Day 5	Olive Phyllo Pies with Honey Syrup	Mediterranean Falafel Salad	Hazelnuts	Sweet and Easy Herb-baked Sweet Potatoes	Strawberries
	2 glasses of water	2 glasses of water	2 glasses of water	1 small glass of red wine	1 glass of water

				1 glass of water	
Day 6	Crispy Pita Bread with Feta Cheese Filling	Greek Rice Spanakokorizo with Spinach	Almonds	Cauliflower Rice with Rotini Pasta and Sausage	Blueberries
	2 glasses of water	2 glasses of water	2 glasses of water	1 small glass of red wine 1 glass of water	1 glass of water
Day 7	Tahini-Feta Toast	Spetzofai Sausage and Peppers	Pistachios	Classic Greek Lemon Roasted Chicken and Potatoes	Apples
	2 glasses of water	2 glasses of water	2 glasses of water	1 small glass of red wine 1 glass of water	1 glass of water

		Week Seven			
	Breakfast	Lunch	Snack	Dinner	Late Night Snack (or dessert)
Quantity	One Serving	One Serving	One Handful	One Serving	As much as you can eat or make into smoothie
Day 1	Spicy Tuna Quesadilla	Cannellini Bean Salad	Pecans	North African Spiced Shrimps with Couscous	Avocado
	2 glasses of water	2 glasses of water	2 glasses of water	1 small glass of red wine 1 glass of water	1 glass of water
Day 2	Mediterranean Breakfast Quinoa	Edgy Veggie Wraps	Dates	One Pan Mediterranean Chicken	Oranges
	2 glasses of water	2 glasses of water	2 glasses of water	1 small glass of red wine 1 glass of water	1 glass of water
Day 3	Low Carb Mediterranean Egg Muffins with Ham	Carrot, Orange & Avocado Salad	Peanuts	Smoky Tempeh Tostadas with Mango Cabbage Slaw	Apples
	2 glasses of water	2 glasses of water	2 glasses of water	1 small glass of red wine 1 glass of water	1 glass of water
Day 4	Greek Goddess Bowl	Panzanella Salad	Pecans	Sweet Potato Noodles with Almond Sauce	Watermelon
	2 glasses of water	2 glasses of water	2 glasses of water	1 small glass of red wine 1 glass of water	1 glass of water
Day 5	Blueberry Oats Bowl	Quinoa & Stir-fried Veggies	Dates	Spiced Carrot and Lentil Soup	Strawberries
	2 glasses of water	2 glasses of water	2 glasses of water	1 small glass of red wine 1 glass of water	1 glass of water
Day 6	Banana Yogurt Pots	Mixed Bean Salad	Peanuts	Mediterranean Chicken Quinoa & Greek Salad	Blueberries
	2 glasses of water	2 glasses of water	2 glasses of water	1 small glass of red wine 1 glass of water	1 glass of water
Day 7	Tomato and Watermelon Salad	Moroccan Chickpea Soup	Pecans	Grilled Vegetables with Bean	Apples

			Mash	
2 glasses of water	2 glasses of water	2 glasses of water	1 small glass of red wine 1 glass of water	1 glass of water

	Week Eight				
	Breakfast	**Lunch**	**Snack**	**Dinner**	**Late Night Snack (or dessert)**
Quantity	One Serving	One Serving	One Handful	One Serving	As much as you can eat or make into smoothie
Day 1	Italian Breakfast Frittata	One Pan Healthy Paella	Cashew Nuts	Israeli Yellow Chicken and Potatoes	Avocado
	2 glasses of water	2 glasses of water	2 glasses of water	1 small glass of red wine 1 glass of water	1 glass of water
Day 2	Italian Breakfast Couscous with Currants	Greek Chicken Zucchini Noodles	Macadamia Nuts	Israeli Green Rice	Oranges
	2 glasses of water	2 glasses of water	2 glasses of water	1 small glass of red wine 1 glass of water	1 glass of water
Day 3	North African Farka (Breakfast Pasta)	Beef Stuffed Acorn Squash	Brazil Nuts	Italian Hot Dish Dinner	Apples
	2 glasses of water	2 glasses of water	2 glasses of water	1 small glass of red wine 1 glass of water	1 glass of water
Day 4	Semolina Pancakes with Honey Butter	Healthy Baked Ziti	Peanuts	Easy Pasta Skillet Dinner	Watermelon
	2 glasses of water	2 glasses of water	2 glasses of water	1 small glass of red wine 1 glass of water	1 glass of water
Day 6	Mediterranean Scrambled Eggs	Cannellini Bean Salad	Macadamia Nuts	Healthy Lasagna	Blueberries

	2 glasses of water	2 glasses of water	2 glasses of water	1 small glass of red wine 1 glass of water	1 glass of water
Day 7	Mediterranean Breakfast Quesadillas	Edgy Veggie Wraps	Brazil Nuts	North African Spiced Carrots	Apples
	2 glasses of water	2 glasses of water	2 glasses of water	1 small glass of red wine 1 glass of water	1 glass of water

MONTH THREE

		Week Nine			
	Breakfast	Lunch	Snack	Dinner	Late Night Snack (or dessert)
Quantity	One Serving	One Serving	One Handful	One Serving	As much as you can eat or make into smoothie
Day 1	Greek Burgers	Mediterranean Hummus Pasta	Cashew Nuts	Honey Lemon Chicken Laps	Avocado
	2 glasses of water	2 glasses of water	2 glasses of water	1 small glass of red wine 1 glass of water	1 glass of water
Day 2	Patsavouropita Cheese and Herb Pie	Greek Kale Quinoa Chicken Salad	Macadamia Nuts	Grilled Chicken Skewers served with Vegetable Salad	Oranges
	2 glasses of water	2 glasses of water	2 glasses of water	1 small glass of red wine 1 glass of water	1 glass of water
Day 3	Sweet Potato and Feta Tart	Pan Roasted Salmon	Brazil Nuts	Cod and Asparagus Bake	Apples
	2 glasses of water	2 glasses of water	2 glasses of water	1 small glass of red wine 1 glass of water	1 glass of water
Day 4	Traditional Greek Feta Cheese Pie	Tabbouleh Salad	Peanuts	Lemon Chicken with Asparagus	Watermelon
	2 glasses of water	2 glasses of water	2 glasses of water	1 small glass of red wine 1 glass of water	1 glass of water
Day 5	Olive Phyllo Pies with Honey Syrup	Mediterranean Falafel Salad	Cashew Nuts	Sweet and Easy Herb-baked	Strawberries

				Sweet Potatoes	
	2 glasses of water	2 glasses of water	2 glasses of water	1 small glass of red wine 1 glass of water	1 glass of water
Day 6	Crispy Pita Bread with Feta Cheese Filling	Greek Rice Spanakokorizo with Spinach	Macadamia Nuts	Cauliflower Rice with Rotini Pasta and Sausage	Blueberries
	2 glasses of water	2 glasses of water	2 glasses of water	1 small glass of red wine 1 glass of water	1 glass of water
Day 7	Tahini-Feta Toast	Spetzofai Sausage and Peppers	Brazil Nuts 2 glasses of water	Classic Greek Lemon Roasted Chicken and Potatoes	Apples
	2 glasses of water	2 glasses of water	2 glasses of water	1 small glass of red wine 1 glass of water	1 glass of water

	Week Ten				
	Breakfast	**Lunch**	**Snack**	**Dinner**	**Late Night Snack (or dessert)**
Quantity	One Serving	One Serving	One Handful	One Serving	As much as you can eat or make into smoothie
Day 1	Greek-Barley Rusks	Roasted Cauliflower with Cheese and Garlic	Pecans	Grilled Honey Harrissa Chicken Skewers served with Garlicky Mint Sauce	Avocado
	2 glasses of water	2 glasses of water	2 glasses of water	1 small glass of red wine 1 glass of water	1 glass of water
Day 2	Baked Olive Oil Croutons	Greek Peas-Arakas Latheros	Dates	Greek-inspired Baked Mac and Cheese	Oranges
	2 glasses of water	2 glasses of water	2 glasses of water	1 small glass of red wine 1 glass of water	1 glass of water
Day 3	Breakfast Shakshukka with Fresh Herbs	Tuscan Tomato and Bread Salad	Peanuts	Greek-styled Juicy Roasted Meatballs	Apples
	2 glasses of water	2 glasses of water	2 glasses of water	1 small glass of red wine 1 glass of water	1 glass of water
Day 4	North African Breakfast Khlea and Egg	Greek Marinated Anchovies	Pecans	Stewed Pork and Greens in Lemon Sauce	Watermelon
	2 glasses of water	2 glasses of water	2 glasses of water	1 small glass of red wine 1 glass of water	1 glass of water
Day 5	Isreali	Pan-roasted	Dates	Greek	Strawberries

	Breakfast Baba Ganoush	Herbs and Garlic Crusted Sardines		Chicken Cooked in Diced Tomato	
	2 glasses of water	2 glasses of water	2 glasses of water	1 small glass of red wine / 1 glass of water	1 glass of water
Day 6	Israeli Breakfast Walnut Hummus	Baked Phyllo Chips	Peanuts	Roasted Veggies Pita Pizza	Blueberries
	2 glasses of water	2 glasses of water	2 glasses of water	1 small glass of red wine / 1 glass of water	1 glass of water
Day 7	Israeli Overnight Breakfast Labane	Mediterranean Chicken Orzo	Pecans	Italian Sheet Pan Eggs with Prosciutto and Artichokes	Apples
	2 glasses of water	2 glasses of water	2 glasses of water	1 small glass of red wine / 1 glass of water	1 glass of water

	Week Eleven				
	Breakfast	Lunch	Snack	Dinner	Late Night Snack (or dessert)
Quantity	One Serving	One Serving	One Handful	One Serving	As much as you can eat or make into smoothie
Day 1	Italian Breakfast Frittata	One Pan Healthy Paella	Pistachios	Israeli Yellow Chicken and Potatoes	Avocado
	2 glasses of water	2 glasses of water	2 glasses of water	1 small glass of red wine 1 glass of water	1 glass of water
Day 2	Italian Breakfast Couscous with Currants	Greek Chicken Zucchini Noodles	Hazelnuts	Israeli Green Rice	Oranges
	2 glasses of water	2 glasses of water	2 glasses of water	1 small glass of red wine 1 glass of water	1 glass of water
Day 3	North African Farka (Breakfast Pasta)	Beef Stuffed Acorn Squash	Almonds	Italian Hot Dish Dinner	Apples
	2 glasses of water	2 glasses of water	2 glasses of water	1 small glass of red wine 1 glass of water	1 glass of water
Day 4	Semolina Pancakes with Honey Butter	Healthy Baked Ziti	Pistachios	Easy Pasta Skillet Dinner	Watermelon
	2 glasses of water	2 glasses of water	2 glasses of water	1 small glass of red wine 1 glass of water	1 glass of water
Day 5	Morrocan Breakfast Msemmen	Mediterranean Bento Bowl	Hazelnuts	Easy Minestrone Soup Dinner	Strawberries
	2 glasses of water	2 glasses of water	2 glasses of water	1 small glass of red wine 1 glass of water	1 glass of water
Day 6	Mediterranean Scrambled	Cannellini Bean Salad	Almonds	Healthy Lasagna	Blueberries

	Eggs				
	2 glasses of water	2 glasses of water	2 glasses of water	1 small glass of red wine 1 glass of water	1 glass of water
Day 7	Mediterranean Breakfast Quesadillas	Edgy Veggie Wraps	Pistachios	North African Spiced Carrots	Apples
	2 glasses of water	2 glasses of water	2 glasses of water	1 small glass of red wine 1 glass of water	1 glass of water

Week Twelve

	Breakfast	Lunch	Snack	Dinner	Late Night Snack(or dessert)
Quantity	One Serving	One Serving	One Handful	One Serving	As much as you can eat or make into smoothie
Day 1	Spicy Tuna Quesadilla	Cannellini Bean Salad	Black Sesame seeds	North African Spiced Shrimps with Couscous	Avocado
	2 glasses of water	2 glasses of water	2 glasses of water	1 small glass of red wine 1 glass of water	1 glass of water
Day 2	Mediterranean Breakfast Quinoa	Edgy Veggie Wraps	Pine nuts	One Pan Mediterranean Chicken	Oranges
	2 glasses of water	2 glasses of water	2 glasses of water	1 small glass of red wine 1 glass of water	1 glass of water
Day 3	Low Carb Mediterranean Egg Muffins with Ham	Carrot, Orange & Avocado Salad	Walnuts	Smoky Tempeh Tostadas with Mango Cabbage Slaw	Apples
	2 glasses of water	2 glasses of water	2 glasses of water	1 small glass of red wine 1 glass of water	1 glass of water
Day 4	Greek Goddess Bowl	Panzanella Salad	Black Sesame seeds	Sweet Potato Noodles with Almond Sauce	Watermelon
	2 glasses of water	2 glasses of water	2 glasses of water	1 small glass of red wine 1 glass of water	1 glass of water
Day 5	Blueberry Oats Bowl	Quinoa & Stir-fried Veggies	Pine nuts	Moussaka	Strawberries
	2 glasses of water	2 glasses of water	2 glasses of water	1 small glass of red wine 1 glass of water	1 glass of water
Day 6	Banana Yogurt Pots	Mixed Bean Salad	Walnuts	Spiced Tomato Baked Eggs	Blueberries
	2 glasses of water	2 glasses of water	2 glasses of water	1 small glass of red wine 1 glass of water	1 glass of water

Day 7	Tomato and Watermelon Salad	Moroccan Chickpea Soup	Black Sesame seeds	Salmon with Potato and Corn Salad	Apples
	2 glasses of water	2 glasses of water	2 glasses of water	1 small glass of red wine 1 glass of water	1 glass of water

Chapter Eight

Mediterranean Diet Shopping List (and Where to Get Stuff From)

Now, note that this shopping list is only for you if you would like to follow the 3 month menu plan. It has an extensive list of all of the items that you'll typically need to prepare all of the meals on the menu plan.

Of course, you don't have to buy all of these items all at once if you cannot afford it. You can shop per meal or per week- whatever works for you.

And of course, you can create your own meal plan to suit your budget and tastes based on the rules of the diet that you have learned.

Bread & Grains	Vegetables	Beans & Legumes
<ul><li>Whole-wheat bread crumbs</li><li>Phyllo (Unleavened dough)</li><li>All-purpose flour</li><li>Whole wheat bread</li><li>Whole grain wheat flour</li><li>Whole wheat pita bread</li><li>Whole grain barley flour</li><li>Whole wheat couscous</li><li>Semolina</li><li>Tortillas</li><li>Quinoa</li><li>Gluten-free Pasta</li></ul>	<ul><li>Sweet Potatoes</li><li>Vine tomatoes</li><li>Green Peppers</li><li>Egg plant</li><li>Red Peppers</li><li>Yellow Peppers</li><li>Green Peppers</li><li>Zucchini</li><li>Asparagus</li><li>Spring Onions</li><li>Cherry Tomatoes</li><li>Jalapeno</li><li>Spinach</li><li>Carrots</li><li>Kale</li><li>Cauliflower</li><li>Potato</li><li>Swiss Chard</li><li>Scallion</li><li>Baby spinach</li></ul>	<ul><li>Garbanzo beans</li><li>Frozen peas</li><li>Sugar snap peas</li><li>Chickpeas</li></ul>

- Farro - Medium grain rice - Whole wheat Orzo Pasta (dried) - Brown rice - Whole wheat Ziti pasta (Chickpea Pasta) - Rotini pasta - Basmati rice - Multigrain bowtie pasta - Gluten-free pasta - Red kidney pasta - Multigrain farfalle pasta - Lasagna noodles - Couscous	- Kale - Celery stalk - Red Cabbage - Lettuce - Summer squash - Acorn squash - Zucchini - Artichoke hearts	
Eggs & Diary	**Herbs & Spices**	**Fruit**
- Eggs - Feta Cheese - Greek Yogurt - Parmesan Cheese - Milk - Ricotta Cheese - Heavy cream - Mozzarella Cheese - Romano cheese - Cream cheese - Tempeh - Almond Milk (unsweetened)	- Onions - Parsley - Black pepper - Dried Oregano - Dried Mint - Mint - Nutmeg - Dill - Tahini - Fresh garlic cloves - Sweet paprika - Ground cumin - Fresh mint - Red pepper flakes - Flat-leaf parsley - Cayenne Pepper - Basil - Parsley - Cinnamon Stick - Fennel - Red Onions - Peppercorns - Dried onion flakes - Saffron threads - Thyme - Fresh sage - Baby Bella Mushrooms - Dried Figs - Garlic powder - Turmeric	- Green Olives - Fresh lemon - Black Olives - Kalamata Olives - Allspice berries - Mangoes - Avocado - Oranges - Apples - Watermelon - Strawberries - Blueberries - Apples

	• Shallots • Tarragon • Capers • Chili powder • Cilantro	
Nuts & Seed	**Meat & Poultry**	**Oils & Fats**
• Black Sesame seeds • Pine nuts • Roasted Walnuts • Walnuts • Pistachios • Hazelnuts • Almonds • Pecans • Dates • Cashew Nuts • Macadamia Nuts • Brazil Nuts • Peanuts	• Ground beef • Khlea (marinated and preserved meat usually made with beef or lamb) • Deli Ham • Shredded Chicken • Sausage • Chicken breasts • Ground turkey • Chicken laps • Sweet Italian Bulk sausage • Pork shoulder • Prosciutto • Italian turkey sausage	• Olive Oil • Unsalted Butter • Coconut Oil • Walnut Oil • Grape seed oil
Fish & Seafood	**Condiments**	**Pantry Essentials**
• Salmon Fillets • Fresh Anchovies • Fresh sardines • Cod fillets • Shrimps	• Herbs de Provence • Lemon zest • Tomato Sauce • Za'atar (Middle Eastern spice mixture made with dried thyme, oregano, marjoram, sumac and toasted sesame seeds) • Canned Tomatoes • Pesto Sauce • Canned Roasted Peppers • Tzatzaki Sauce (Middle Eastern Sauce made with salted strained yogurt and a blend of herbs and spices) • Greek salad dressing • Falafel mix • Trader Joe's Mediterranean-style Salad Kit • Chicken broth	• Salt • Honey • Dry yeast • Dried Currants • Dark brown sugar • Baking Powder • Vanilla extract • Sea salt • Maple Syrup • Hummus • Red wine vinegar • Kosher Salt • Fresh mustard • White wine • Bay leaves • Agave Nectar • Apple Cider Vinegar • Hot sauce • Liquid smoke • Fresh lime juice

	<ul><li>Canned chopped tomatoes</li><li>Harrisa (Tunisian hot chili pepper paste)</li><li>Chicken Bouillon powder</li><li>Chili flakes</li><li>Ras El Hanout Sauce</li><li>Soy Sauce</li><li>Dijon Mustard</li><li>Salsa</li></ul>	

Where to Get Mediterranean Diet Ingredients From

What's a Mediterranean diet without some specialized ingredients and condiments straight from the Mediterranean?

You're going to come across some unfamiliar ingredients in the recipes and naturally, you'll wonder how to get them.

Some of these ingredients have the 'Western substitutes' and I've indicated the substitutes where applicable but for those without substitutes or if you would love to follow the recipes religiously, you can get the ingredients easily from:

- **Amazon**: Use the search bar on Amazon to search for the ingredients and you'll be able to find most of them on sale. The Mediterranean diet is growing increasingly popular so many online stores now stock Mediterranean-themed condiments and food supplies.

- **Middle Eastern Stores**: If there are Middle Eastern Stores in your cities, like Persian, Turkish or Israeli stores, you'll be able to find many of these ingredients there.

- **Online Stores**: You'll also be able to find a lot of ingredients in Mediterranean online stores like igourmet.com, persianbasket.com, and kalamala.com.

Breakfast Recipes

Blueberry Oats Bowl

Ingredients
Servings 2

- 400 Ml of water
- 1 teaspoon of honey
- ⅔ cup (60g) of porridge oats
- 1 ¾ cups (175g) of blueberries
- ⅗ cup (160g) of Greek yogurt

Cooking Directions

- Pour the water in a small pot placed over medium heat and add oats.
- Stir the oats continuously for 2 minutes.
- Divide yogurt into three portions and add one portion to the oats. Stir and remove from heat.
- Place another saucepan over heat and add the honey, blueberries, and a tablespoon of water. Poach until the berries are tender.
- Serve oats topped with the poached berries and the remaining Greek yogurt.

Banana Yogurt Pots

Ingredients
Servings 2

- ⅞ (225g) cup of Greek yogurt
- 2 tablespoons (15g) of toasted and chopped walnuts
- 2 bananas (sliced into chunks)

Cooking Directions
- Pour the Greek yogurt in the bottom of a glass cup or jar.
- Add a layer of banana on top of the yogurt.
- Add another layer of Greek yogurt and repeat the layers until you have no yogurt or bananas left.
- Top with toasted and chopped walnuts.
- Serve.

Tomato and Watermelon Salad

Ingredients
Servings 2

- 1 tablespoon of olive oil
- ⅔ cup (100g) of crumbled feta cheese
- 1 tablespoon of red wine vinegar
- ½ watermelon (cut into chunks)
- ¼ teaspoon of chili flakes
- ⅝ cup (120g) of chopped tomatoes
- 1 tablespoon of chopped mint

Cooking Directions

- Combine olive oil, chili flakes, vinegar, and mint in a jar. Cover it up and shake the jar vigorously to mix the ingredients.
- Combine watermelon and chopped tomatoes in a salad bowl.
- Add dressing the olive oil dressing from the jar and toss to coat.
- Top with crumbled feta cheese
- Serve.

Greek Burgers

Ingredients
Servings 5

- 1 lbs. of ground beef chucks
- 1 egg
- 4 tablespoons of breadcrumbs
- 1 small onion (grated)
- 2 tablespoons of fresh parsley
- ½ teaspoon of salt
- Freshly ground pepper
- 1 teaspoon of dried oregano
- 1 teaspoon of dried mint

Cooking Directions

- Pour your beef into a large bowl and add all the other ingredients.
- Use your hands to knead the beef until it is well mixed.
- Place in your refrigerator for 1 hour to marinate.
- Ten minutes before you start your cooking, remove the beef from the refrigerator and form 5 patties from it.
- Place a grill pan over heat and let it heat up.
- Add your patties to cook for 4 minutes.
- Serve with lemon juice squeezed over it.

Patsavouropita Cheese and Herb Pie

Ingredients
Servings 8

- 2 eggs
- 7 ounces of crumbled feta cheese
- 2 tablespoons of Greek yoghurt
- 1/4 cup of grated parmesan cheese
- 6 sheets of Phyllo
- ¼ teaspoon of nutmeg
- ½ cup of chopped mint
- Salt and pepper to taste

Cooking Directions

- Preheat your oven to 350 F.
- Take 1 phyllo dough sheet and spread it on a work surface. Spray it lightly with olive oil.
- Scrunch the phyllo like a curtain and place it in the base of a 12 by 8 inch baking pan.
- Repeat with the remaining phyllo until the base of your pan is completely covered.
- One scrunched sheet should be placed next to the other.
- Place the pan in the oven to bake for 5 minutes
- While it is baking, combine eggs, feta cheese, yoghurt, nutmeg, Parmesan cheese, pepper, mint, and a tablespoon of olive oil in a large bowl. Mix well to combine.
- Remove the pan from the oven and pour mixture over the phyllo.
- Sprinkle some crumbs of feta cheese on the surface and drizzle with a teaspoon of olive oil.
- Return to the oven and bake for 30 minutes.
- Remove, slice and serve.

Sweet Potato and Feta Tart

Ingredients
Servings 8

- 2 lbs. Sweet potatoes (chopped into ½ inch cubes)
- ¼ cup of milk
- ¼ cup of olive oil
- 1 tablespoon of grated Parmesan cheese
- 7 ounces crumbled Feta Cheese
- 2 eggs
- 6 sheets of Phyllo
- 1 tablespoon of Herbs de Provence
- 1 tablespoon of Parmesan (grated)
- Freshly ground pepper
- ½ teaspoon of salt
- 1 medium onions (diced)

Cooking Directions

- Preheat your oven to 400 F.
- Pour the chopped sweet potatoes into a bowl and drizzle with 1 ½ tablespoon of olive oil until the potato is well coated.
- Pour the mixture in a pan and place in the oven to roast for 25 minutes.
- Remove and set aside.
- Place a saucepan over medium heat and add 2 teaspoons of olive oil to heat up.
- Add onions and sauté until translucent.
- Combine feta, herbs de Provence, milk, 1 teaspoon of salt, eggs, freshly ground pepper, and 1 1/2 tablespoon of olive oil to a bowl and mix.
- Now, add the onions and sweet potatoes. Mix everything together very well.
- Spray a 10-inch tart pan lightly with olive oil and arrange the Phyllo in the pan.
- Brush the surface of each Phyllo sheet with olive oil.

- Pour the potato mixture inside the pan. Use a spatula to spread evenly.
- Sprinkle parmesan over it.
- Cover the pan with aluminum foil and place in the oven to bake for 20 minutes.
- Allow it to cool up then slice and serve.

Traditional Greek Feta Cheese Pie

Ingredients
Servings 12

- 3 eggs
- 17 ounces of feta cheese
- 1 tablespoon of olive oil
- 9 ounces of fresh ricotta cheese
- 12 Phyllo sheets
- 2 tablespoons of fresh dill (chopped)
- 3 tablespoons of fresh mint (minced)
- Black sesame seeds
- Freshly ground black pepper
- Salt to taste

Cooking Directions

- Pre-heat your oven to 350 F
- Spray a 9 by 13 inch casserole dish with olive oil or cooking spray.
- Crumble feta cheese in a large bowl with a fork, and add the ricotta cheese. Crumble ricotta cheese as well.
- Add pepper, dill and mint. Continue to mix until everything is well incorporated.
- In another small bowl, break your eggs and beat it.
- Add the previous cheese mixture into the egg mixture and whisk it well.
- Add a tablespoon of olive oil and continue to whisk it very well.

- Spread one Phyllo sheet on the bottom of a baking pan. Brush with olive oil.
- Spread the cheese mixture on the Phyllo sheet and cover it with a second Phyllo sheet.
- Repeat the process until you have multiple layers of Phyllo sheets with cheese mixture in the middle.
- Top with sesame seeds and a sprinkle of water.
- Now, place in the oven to bake for 40 minutes.
- Allow it to cool up, slice and serve.

Olive Phyllo Pies with Honey Syrup

Ingredients

Servings 16

- 3 pounds of Kataifi Phyllo
- Two tablespoons of olive oil
- 3 cups of olives (chopped)
- 1 teaspoon of lemon zest
- 1 tablespoon of dried oregano
- Freshly ground pepper
- 2 onions (thinly sliced)

Cooking Directions

- Place a pan over medium heat and add olive oil to heat up.
- Add onions and sauté for 20 minutes until caramelized.
- Add olives to the caramelized onions, stir before adding lemon zest, oregano, pepper, and salt to taste. Stir, then remove from heat and set aside to cool.
- Separate your Phyllo into 16 sections. Each section should be 6 inches long and 2 inches wide.
- Cover up the Phyllo with a damp towel for a few minutes.
- Remove the towel and brush the phyllo with olive oil.
- Pour 1 tablespoon of filling on each section and roll It tightly.
- Place your rolls in a pan and brush with olive oil again.
- Place in the oven and bake for 20 minutes.
- Serve drizzled with honey.

Crispy Pita Bread with Feta Cheese Filling

Ingredients
Servings 12

- 3 ounces of feta cheese
- 2 cups of all-purpose four
- 3 tablespoons of olive oil
- Extra olive oil for frying
- 2 tablespoons of chopped mint
- 1 teaspoon of salt

Cooking Directions

- Pour the all-purpose flour in a bowl and mix with salt, 3 tablespoons of olive oil, and ½ cup of water. Form dough.
- Place the dough on a flat surface and knead it until it is soft and stretchy.
- Cut it into 12 pieces and roll each piece into a ball.
- Pour feta cheese into a bowl and mash it into a paste.
- Add mint to the cheese, mash and mix.
- Scoop ½ teaspoon of feta cheese and spread it on each ball of dough.
- Fold the dough in so the cheese mixture sits in the middle of each ball of dough.
- Pour olive oil in a frying plan placed over medium heat. Olive oil should be just enough for frying the dough.
- Put the pita balls inside the pan in batches and fry for 1 minute. Flip and fry again for another minute.
- Repeat until you've fried the entire batch.
- Serve immediately.

Tahini-Feta Toast

Ingredients
Servings 2

- 2 teaspoons of crumbled feta
- 2 slices of whole wheat bread
- Juice of 1 lemon
- 2 slices of toasted whole wheat bread
- 1 tablespoon of tahini
- Pepper to taste
- Pine nuts

Cooking Directions

- Pour tahini and lemon juice in a bowl and mix with 1 teaspoon of water until it forms a thick peanut butter-like paste.
- Spread the paste on your toast and sprinkle with pepper, pine nuts, and crumbled feta.
- Serve.

Greek-Barley Rusks

Ingredients
Servings 4

- 0.2 ounces of whole grain wheat flour
- 2 ½ teaspoons of dry yeast
- 0.2 ounces of whole grain barley flour
- ½ teaspoon of sugar
- ½ teaspoon of salt

Cooking Directions

- Preheat your oven to 350F.
- Pour the yeast in a large bowl and add 1 ½ cup of warm water.
- Add sugar and set aside for 10 minutes.
- When you start to see bubbles on the surface of the water, add the flours and salt. Mix together to form dough.
- Knead the dough for about 10 minutes.
- Cover up and let it sit for a few minutes.
- Cut dough up into small round disks.
- Cover up and let it sit for a few minutes so the dough can rise again.
- Arrange the disks on a baking sheet.
- Bake in your oven for 2 hours until completely dried.
- Serve.

Baked Olive Oil Croutons

Ingredients
Servings 3

- 1/3 cups of olive oil
- 3 cups of cubed baguette or bread
- Pepper and salt to taste
- 2 garlic cloves (minced)

Cooking Directions

- Preheat your oven to 350F.
- Place a saucepan over medium heat and add a dash of olive oil to heat up.
- Add minced garlic and sauté for 2 minutes.
- Pour the bread cubes into a large dish and add sautéed garlic. Mix well.
- Line a baking pan with aluminum foil.
- Pour everything into the baking pan and spread.
- Drizzle with olive oil.
- Place in the oven to bake for 10 minutes.
- Sprinkle with salt and pepper.
- Serve or store in an airtight container for later consumption. These olive oil croutons can hold up for about 2 weeks.

Breakfast Shakshukka with Fresh Herbs

Ingredients
Servings 6

- 2 green peppers (chopped)
- 6 ripe vine tomatoes (chopped)
- ½ cup of tomato sauce
- 6 large eggs
- 3 tablespoons of olive oil
- 1 teaspoon of sweet paprika
- 2 garlic cloves (chopped)
- ½ teaspoon of ground cumin
- Salt and pepper to taste
- ¼ cup of fresh parsley (chopped)
- ¼ cup of fresh mint (chopped)
- One pinch of red pepper flakes
- 1 teaspoon of sugar

Cooking Directions

- Place a large skillet over medium heat and add the olive oil to heat up.
- Add garlic and onions.
- Add all your peppers, herbs (except parsley and mint), spices, and a pinch of salt. Cook for 10 minutes.
- Add tomato sauce, vine tomatoes and your sugar. Stir and allow simmer for 10 minutes.
- Adjust seasoning.
- Make 6 holes in the pan.
- Crack an egg into each hole.
- Cover the skillet and let it cook until the egg white sets.
- Sprinkle with fresh mint and parsley.
- Serve with pita bread.

North African Breakfast Khlea and Egg

Ingredients
Servings 2

- 6 eggs
- 4 tablespoons of Khlea (marinated meat)
- 1 tablespoon of heavy cream
- A pinch of salt
- A pinch of cumin
- Fresh parsley(finely chopped)

Cooking Directions

- Crack eggs into a bowl and beat it with a fork.
- Add salt and beat with eggs.
- Place a tangine or frying pan over medium heat and add the khlea. Wait for 5 minutes or until the fat melts.
- Scoop about 2 tablespoons of the fat out and discard it.
- Pour the eggs into the khlea.
- Let it cook for 30 seconds.
- Scramble.
- Sprinkle the remaining herbs on it.
- Serve.

Isreali Breakfast Baba Ganoush

Ingredients
Servings 4

- 1 tablespoon of extra virgin olive oil
- 2 eggplants
- 2 tablespoons of flat-leaf parsley (chopped)
- 1 clove of garlic (crushed),
- ¾ teaspoons of salt
- ¼ teaspoon of cumin
- 1/3 cup of tahini
- Pinch of cayenne pepper

Cooking Directions

- Preheat your oven to 450F.
- Cut eggplants into halves lengthwise.
- Place the eggplants on a baking tray with the cut side facing up.
- Brush with olive oil and roast in your oven for 35 minutes.
- Set aside to cool.
- Use a fork to scoop out the fleshy part of your roasted eggplant into a bowl.
- Mash and mix with all other ingredients.
- Discard the flesh.
- Serve.

Israeli Breakfast Walnut Hummus

Ingredients
Servings 2

- ¼ cup of olive oil
- ½ cup of roasted walnuts
- Juice of 1 lemon
- 2 cups of Garbanzo beans (cooked)
- 2 garlic cloves
- 1 tablespoon of Za'atar (can substitute with paprika)

Cooking Directions

- Pour roasted walnuts in a food processor and process until sandy (not smooth).
- Add the garbanzo beans, lemon juice, 1 clove of garlic, and a tablespoon of oil. Process until smooth whilst adding a little bit of water at a time until you get a creamy texture.
- Adjust for seasoning.
- Serve drizzled with paprika and olive oil.

Israeli Overnight Breakfast Labane

Ingredients
Servings 1

- 1 cup of Greek Yoghurt
- 1 teaspoon of salt
- 1 teaspoon of olive oil
- 1 teaspoon of Za'atar

Cooking Directions

- Add salt to your Greek Yoghurt and stir.
- Place a mesh strainer over a bowl and cover with saran wrap.
- Let it sit in your refrigerator overnight.
- Remove from the refrigerator and discard the whey.
- Pour the strained yoghurt in a shallow serving bowl and add all the other ingredients.
- Serve.

Italian Breakfast Frittata

Ingredients
Servings 8

- 6 eggs
- ¼ cup of Parmesan cheese
- ¼ cup of mozzarella cheese
- 3 cups of mixed boiled veggies (chopped tomatoes, chopped peppers, zucchini, eggplant, asparagus)
- 1 tablespoon of olive oil
- Ground black pepper and salt to taste
- 2 tablespoons of mixed fresh herbs(oregano, parsley, basil)

Cooking Directions

- Place a pan over medium heat and add olive oil to heat up.
- Add vegetables and sauté until softened.
- Crack eggs and whisk.
- Add all the herbs and seasonings and continue to whisk.
- Spoon egg mixture on top of the veggies and stir once so the veggies and eggs are well mixed.
- Lift the edges of the egg frequently with a fork so it doesn't burn, and so the liquid from the veggies can stay at the bottom of the pan.
- Cook until everything is firm.
- Set your broiler to low and broil for 2 minutes.
- Cut up and serve.

Italian Breakfast Couscous with Currants

Ingredients
Servings 4

- 4 teaspoons of butter (melted)
- ¼ cup of dried currants
- 3 cups of 1% low-fat milk
- 1 2-inch cinnamon stick
- 1 cup of whole wheat couscous
- 1/4 teaspoon of salt
- 6 tablespoons of dark brown sugar

Cooking Directions

- Place a large saucepan over medium heat.
- Pour milk in the pan and add cinnamon sticks.
- Let it heat up for 3 minutes but make sure it doesn't burn.
- Add all the other ingredients except sugar and butter, and stir.
- Cover it up and let it cook for 15 minutes.
- Discard cinnamon stick.
- Serve with brown sugar and melted butter added to each bowl.

North African Farka (Breakfast Pasta)

Ingredients
Servings 8

- 2 ½ cups of couscous
- ¼ cup of olive oil
- ½ cup of honey
- 1 ½ cup of toasted nuts mix (walnuts, pistachios, hazelnuts, almonds), (chopped)

Cooking Directions

- Preheat your oven to 350F.
- Place a heavy saucepan over medium heat and add 2 2/3 cups of water in it.
- Add olive oil and sugar: bring to a boil.
- Whilst it's boiling, stir continuously so that the sugar dissolves.
- Pour couscous in a bowl and pour the sugar mixture over it.
- Add the chopped nuts and use a fork to fluff it.
- Pour everything in a small baking dish.
- Bake for 20 minutes.
- Serve.

Semolina Pancakes with Honey Butter

Ingredients
Servings 4

- 3 1/2 cups of fine semolina
- 2 tablespoons of plain flour
- 1 teaspoon of baking powder
- 2 teaspoons of dried yeast
- 1/3 cups of honey
- 1/3 cups of unsalted butter

Cooking Directions

- Add semolina, plain flour, baking powder, and dry yeast to a food processor.
- Add 3 cups of water and process to form batter.
- Pour in a bowl and cover with a tea towel. Set aside for 45 minutes.
- Place a frying pan over medium heat and a dash of olive oil.
- Scoop ½ cup of patter into the hot pan and when bubbles start to form on the surface of the pan, flip and cook for 2 minutes.
- Repeat until you've made all the batter into pancakes.
- Make your honey milk by adding honey and milk to your food processor and process.
- Serve pancakes with honey milk drizzled over it.

Moroccan Breakfast Msemmen

Ingredients
Servings 6

- 1 cup of semolina flour
- 1 ½ cup of vegetable oil
- ¼ cup of soft butter (unsalted)
- ¼ teaspoon of yeast
- 3 ½ cups of all-purpose flour
- 2 teaspoons of salt
- 2 teaspoons of sugar

Cooking Directions

- Combine semolina flour, all-purpose flour, and yeast in a bowl and mix.
- Add 1 ½ cup of water to the flour mix to form dough.
- The dough should not be too sticky to handle but should be soft enough. You can add more flour to it becomes too sticky.
- Knead the dough for 10 minutes.
- Divide the sough into golf-sized balls.
- Mix the butter and oil together in a separate bowl.
- Take one ball of dough, rub some of the oil and butter mixture on your hands and flatten the ball slowly into a thin flat layer.
- Rub some of the butter and oil mixture to the surface and fold the flattened dough into thirds.
- Add more butter and oil mixture and sprinkle some more semolina flour on the surface.
- Fold the dough again into thirds so you end up with a small square of dough.
- Repeat the process with the rest of your dough balls.
- Place a skillet over medium heat and add a tablespoon of vegetable oil to the pan to heat up.
- Now, oil your hands and start flattening the dough so it's very thin but remains in that square shape.

- Place in the skillet and fry until golden brown.
- Serve.

Mediterranean Scrambled Eggs

Ingredients
Servings 2

- 4 Eggs
- 1 tablespoon of olive oil
- ¼ teaspoon of oregano
- 1 yellow pepper (diced)
- 1 tablespoon of capers
- 2 tablespoons of black olives (sliced)
- 2 spring onions (sliced)
- 8 cherry tomatoes (quartered)
- Black pepper to taste
- Fresh parsley (topping)

Cooking Directions

- Place a pan over heat and add oil to heat up.
- Add chopped spring onions and diced peppers. Cover the pan and sauté for 2 minutes.
- Add quartered tomatoes, capers, and olives. Cook for 1 minute.
- Crack eggs into the pan and scramble with a spatula.
- Add black pepper and oregano. Continue to stir until eggs are well cooked.
- Serve topped with fresh parsley.

Mediterranean Breakfast Quesadillas

Ingredients
Servings 1

- ½ tomato slices
- 1 tablespoon +1 teaspoon of olive oil
- 2 eggs
- Handful of basil
- ¼ cup of mozzarella cheese
- Pepper and salt to taste

Cooking Directions

- Place a pan over heat and add olive oil to heat up.
- Crack eggs into a bowl and whisk.
- Pour whisked eggs into pan, add salt and pepper to taste, and scramble lightly.
- Spread scrambled eggs on ½ of a tortilla.
- Spread mozzarella cheese, sliced tomatoes, and basil on top.
- Fold tortilla.
- Place a pan over heat and grease the pan with the teaspoon of olive oil.
- Toast tortilla in the pan until all sides turn golden brown.
- Slice and serve.

Spicy Tuna Quesadilla

Ingredients
Servings 2

- 1/3 cup of shredded cheese
- ½ cup of tuna (drained)
- 2 tablespoons of olive oil
- 1 small tomato (chopped)
- 1 teaspoon of dry basil
- 1 garlic clove (minced)
- 1 ½ tablespoon of tomato paste
- 1 green onion (chopped)
- ½ teaspoon of crushed red pepper
- 1 jalapeno (chopped)
- Tortilla

Cooking Directions

- Add drained tuna to a bowl and add tomato paste, crushed red pepper, tomatoes, garlic, green onions, basil, and a tablespoon of olive oil. Mix everything together to make a chunky sauce.
- Spread the mixture on top of half of a tortilla.
- Add shredded cheese on top and fold in half.
- Grease a saucepan with a teaspoon of olive oil.
- Toast folded tortillas in the pan until all sides turn golden brown.
- Slice and serve.

Mediterranean Breakfast Quinoa

Ingredients
Servings 4

- 2 tablespoons of honey
- ¼ cup of raw almonds (chopped)
- 5 dried apricots (finely chopped)
- 1 teaspoon of ground cinnamon
- 1 teaspoon of vanilla extract
- 1 cup of quinoa
- 1 teaspoon of sea salt
- 2 cups of milk

Cooking Directions

- Place a skillet over medium heat and toast the almonds in in for 4 minutes. Remove and set aside.
- Add quinoa and cinnamon to a saucepan placed over medium heat and add milk and sea salt. Stir and bring to a boil.
- Reduce heat to low and let it simmer for 15 minutes.
- Add honey, vanilla, apricots, dates, and half of your toasted almonds. Stir.
- Serve topped with the rest of your almonds.

Low Carb Mediterranean Egg Muffins with Ham

Ingredients
Servings 6

- 1/3 cup of fresh spinach (minced)
- 9 slices of deli ham (deli cut)
- 1 ½ tablespoons of pesto sauce
- ½ cup of roasted peppers (canned, sliced)
- A pinch of salt
- A pinch of pepper
- 5 large eggs
- ¼ cup of crumbled feta cheese
- Fresh basil

Cooking Directions
- Preheat your oven to 400F.
- Spray 6 muffin tins with cooking spray.
- Line the bottom of each tin with 1 ½ piece of ham.
- Add some roasted peppers to the bottom of each tin.
- Add a tablespoon of minced spinach to each tin.
- Add ½ tablespoon of crumbled feta cheese to each pan.
- Crack eggs into a bowl and whisk.
- Add pepper and salt to the eggs and continue to whisk.
- Make a hole in the middle of each muffin tin to make room for the egg mixture.
- Divide the mixture amongst the muffin tins.
- Bake for 15 minutes.
- Scoop egg muffins out of each tin and serve garnished with fresh basil and ¼ teaspoon of pesto sauce.

Greek Goddess Bowl

Ingredients
Servings 2

- 1 tablespoon of spice blend (any)
- 1 15-ounce can of chickpeas (rinsed, drained and towel-dried)
- ¼ teaspoon of sea salt
- 1 tablespoon of coconut oil
- 1 tablespoon of maple syrup
- 1 medium carrot (sliced thinly)
- ¾ cup of Tzatzaki sauce
- 1 medium cucumber (sliced thinly)
- 1 cup of chopped parsley
- 1/2 cup of cherry tomatoes
- ½ cup of kalamata olives (chopped)

Cooking Directions

- Preheat oven to 375F.
- Spray a baking sheet with cooking spray.
- Pour chickpeas into a mixing bowl and add coconut oil, maple syrup, spice blend, and salt to taste. Toss to combine.
- Pour chickpeas in a baking sheet and toast in the oven for 20 minutes or until chickpeas turn golden brown and crispy.
- Divide tzatzaki amongst serving bowls.
- Top with toasted chickpeas.
- Garnish with fresh lemon juice.

LUNCH RECIPES

Cannellini Bean Salad

Ingredients
Servings 2

- 3 cups (600g) of cannellini beans
- Small bunch of basil (torn)
- ⅜ cup (70g) of cherry tomatoes (halved)
- ½ tablespoon of red wine vinegar
- ½ red onion (thinly sliced)

Cooking Directions

- Rinse and drain the beans.
- Add tomatoes to the beans.
- Add vinegar and onions.
- Toss to combine.
- Season, then top with basil.
- Serve.

Edgy Veggie Wraps

Ingredients
Servings 2

- 2 tablespoons of hummus
- ½ cup (100g) of cherry tomato
- ¼ cup (50g) of feta cheese
- 1 cucumber
- 2 large wholemeal tortilla wraps
- 6 kalamata olives

Cooking Directions

- Chop the tomatoes.
- Cut the cucumber into sticks.
- Split the olives and remove the stones.
- Heat up the tortillas.
- Combine cucumber, tomatoes and olives.
- Spread hummus over tortillas and add the veggies on top.
- Serve.

Carrot, Orange & Avocado Salad

Ingredients
Servings 2

- 1 tablespoon of olive oil
- 1 orange (Juice plus zest)
- 1 avocado (Stoned, peeled and sliced)
- 1 ½ cups (35g) of rocket / arugula
- 2 carrots (halved lengthways and sliced with a peeler)

Cooking Directions

- Cut one of the oranges into four segments.
- Put the orange segments into a bowl and add rocket, carrots and avocado.
- Squeeze orange juice in the bowl and whisk everything together.
- Add oil and zest and continue to whisk.
- Season to taste.
- Serve.

Panzanella Salad

Ingredients
Servings 2

- Small handful of basil leaves
- 2 cups (400g) of tomatoes
- 1 tablespoon of red wine vinegar
- 1 garlic clove (crushed)
- 2 tablespoons of olive oil
- 1 tablespoon of capers (drained and rinsed)
- 2 slices of brown bread
- 1 ripe avocado (stoned, peeled and chopped)
- 1 small red onion (very thinly sliced)

Cooking Directions

- Chop tomatoes and add to a bowl.
- Add capers, onions, garlic, avocado and seasoning. Mix everything together.
- Cut bread into chunks. Add bread chunks to a bowl.
- Drizzle half of the vinegar and half of the olive oil over the bread chunks.
- Add basil leaves and tomatoes mixture on top.
- Drizzle with the rest of the oil and vinegar.
- Serve.

Quinoa & Stir-fried Veggies

Ingredients
Servings 2

- Juice ½ lemon
- ⅗ cup (100g) quinoa
- 1 teaspoon of tomato purée
- 3 tablespoons of olive oil
- ½ cup (100ml) of vegetable stock
- ¼ cup (50g) of tomatoes
- 2 carrots (cut into thin sticks)
- 1 broccoli head (cut into small florets)
- 1 ⅔ cups (150g) sliced leek

Cooking Directions

- Cook quinoa according to instructions on the package. Drain and set aside.
- Place a pan over heat and add 3 tablespoons of oil.
- Sauté garlic in the oil for a minute.
- Add carrots, broccoli, and leeks. Stir-fry for 2 minutes.
- Add stock, tomatoes and tomato puree and stir everything together. Let it cook for 3 minutes.
- Add drained quinoa to the pan and toss.
- Drizzle the rest of the lemon juice and the remaining oil over it. Toss to combine.
- Serve.

Mixed Bean Salad

Ingredients
Servings 2

- ⅔ cups (100g) of crumbled feta cheese
- 2 spring onions (thinly sliced on the diagonal)
- ½ teaspoon of red wine vinegar
- Handful of Kalamata black olives
- ⅘ cups (145g) jar of artichoke heart in oil
- ¾ cup (150g) of tomatoes (quartered)
- 1 cup (200g) of cannellini beans (drained and rinsed)
- ½ tablespoon of sundried tomato paste

Cooking Directions

- Scoop out 2 tablespoons of artichokes oil, then drain the rest.
- Combine the 2 tablespoons of artichokes oil with vinegar and dried tomato paste. Stir until smooth.
- Season to taste.
- Now, chop the artichokes and add to a bowl.
- Add olives, tomatoes, cannellini beans, half of the feta cheese and spring onions. Stir to combine.
- Add artichoke oil mix and stir.
- Serve topped with crumbled feta cheese.

Moroccan Chickpea Soup

Ingredients
Servings 2

- 1 tablespoon of olive oil
- Zest and juice of ½ lemon
- ½ medium onion (chopped)
- ¼ cup (50g) of frozen broad beans
- 1 celery sticks (chopped)
- 1 teaspoon of ground cumin
- 1 cup (200g can) of chickpeas (rinsed and drained)
- 1 cup (200g can) of chopped tomatoes
- 1¼ cups (300ml) of hot vegetable stock
- Bread & coriander to serve

Cooking Directions

- Place a pan over low heat and add the oil.
- Add celery and onions and fry for 10 minutes until soft.
- Add cumin and stir-fry for one minute more.
- Increase heat to medium and add tomatoes, stock, black pepper and chickpeas. Let it simmer for 8 minutes.
- Add lemon juice and broad beans. Let it cook for 2 minutes.
- Serve topped with coriander and lemon zest.

Mediterranean Hummus Pasta

Ingredients
Servings 6

- 1 cup of hummus
- ½ cup of walnuts
- 10 ounces of gluten-free pasta
- ½ cup of olives
- 5 cloves of garlic (minced)
- Salt and pepper to taste

Cooking Directions

- Cook pasta according to the instructions on the package.
- Drain cooked pasta and set aside.
- Place a saucepan over medium heat and add the hummus.
- Pour 1/3 cup of water in the saucepan and add olives, walnuts, minced garlic, salt and pepper. Stir and cook for 10 minutes.
- Add cooked pasta and mix.
- Serve.

Greek Kale Quinoa Chicken Salad

Ingredients
Servings 2

- 1 cup of quinoa (cooked)
- 4 cups of kale (chopped)
- ¼ cup of Greek Salad dressing
- 1 ½ cups of shredded chicken (cooked)
- ¼ cup of roasted red peppers (sliced}

Cooking Directions

- Combine kale, quinoa, shredded chicken, and roasted red peppers in a salad bowl and toss.
- Add Greek salad dressing and mix well.
- Serve.

Pan Roasted Salmon

Ingredients
Servings 4

- 1 medium-sized fennel bulb (cored and sliced thinly)
- 4.5 ounces salmon fillets with skin on
- 1 cup of cherry tomatoes
- 3 tablespoons of olive oil
- Mediterranean Rub

Cooking Directions

- First, make your Mediterranean rub by combining ¼ teaspoon of sea salt, 1 teaspoon of basil leaves, ½ teaspoon of rosemary, ½ teaspoon of oregano, and 1 teaspoon of garlic powder.
- Place your fillets on a tray with the skin side facing downwards.
- Sprinkle 2 tablespoonsful of the Mediterranean rub all over the fillets.
- Add 2 tablespoons of olive oil to the remaining Mediterranean rub and stir.
- Add cherry tomatoes and fennel to the mixture and stir.
- Place a large-sized non-stick skillet over medium heat and add the rest of your olive oil. Let it heat up for a few seconds.
- Add salmon to the pan with the skin side facing up.
- Cook for 5 minutes.
- Add the fennel spice mixture to the pan, stir and flip the fillets over.
- Cook for 5 minutes or until the fish is cooked through.
- Serve.

Tabbouleh Salad

Ingredients
Servings 4

- 1/3 cup of red onion (diced)
- 2 tablespoons of extra virgin olive oil
- 5 cups of fresh parsley (chopped)
- 1 large red bell pepper
- Juice of 1 medium-sized lemon
- Sea salt and black pepper to taste

Cooking Directions

- Combine parsley, bell pepper, and onion in a salad bowl. Mix.
- Add olive oil, lemon juice, pepper and salt. Toss to combine.
- Serve.

Mediterranean Falafel Salad

Ingredients
Servings 4

- 1 8.8 ounce bag of 10-minute Farro
- 1 16 ounce bag of Falafel mix
- 1 12.95 ounce bag of Organic Mediterranean Style Salad Kit

Cooking Directions

- Preheat your oven to 350F.
- Follow the instructions on the box of falafel and use it to make a double batch of falafel. Set dough aside.
- Place a large pot of water over heat and bring to a boil.
- Cook Farro in the boiling pot of water or according to the instructions on the package.
- Once faro is cooked, drain and pour drained faro on a rimmed baking sheet. Spread it.
- Place the baking sheet in your refrigerator to cool.
- Form patties with the falalfel dough.
- Place patties on a baking sheet lined with parchment paper and place in your oven.
- Bake for 25 minutes until it turns golden brown and puffed.
- Divide the salad kit amongst the serving dishes.
- Top with baked falafel and cooked faro.
- Serve.

Greek Rice Spanakokorizo with Spinach

Ingredients
Servings 4

- 1 tablespoon of tomato paste
- Juice of 1/2 lemon
- 2 1/2 tablespoons of olive oil
- 1/3 cups of medium grain rice
- 1 Pound of fresh spinach
- 1 onion (chopped)
- 1 teaspoon of dried mint
- Salt and pepper to taste
- 2 tablespoons of chopped dill

Cooking Directions

- Combine lemon juice, spinach, and a teaspoon of olive oil in a large pot to wilt.
- Set aside to drain.
- Place another pot over medium heat and add onions. Add the rest of your olive oil. Sauté until onions are soft.
- Add your spinach, dry mint, and 2/3 cups of warm water to the pot stir.
- Cover the pot and bring to a boil.
- Add rice to the boiling pot of water.
- Add salt and pepper to taste.
- Cover the pot and let it simmer for 20 minutes or until the rice is very soft.
- Serve with a squeeze of lemon juice and olive oil drizzled over it.

Spetzofai Sausage and Peppers

Ingredients
Servings 2

- 12 ounces of tomatoes (chopped)
- 3 ounces of sausage (sliced)
- 2 red bell peppers (sliced)
- 2 green bell peppers (sliced)
- ½ cup of olive oil
- 2 teaspoons of dried oregano
- Freshly ground black pepper
- 1/8 teaspoon of salt
- 2 garlic cloves

Cooking Directions

- Place a large pan over medium heat and add olive oil to heat up
- Add sausage and peppers to the pan and sauté for 5 minutes
- Add garlic and salt and sauté for 1 minute more.
- Add tomatoes and stir well.
- Reduce heat and allow to simmer for 20 minutes
- Add a little bit of hot water while it is simmering
- Turn off the heat and add pepper and oregano.
- Serve with pasta or bread.

Roasted Cauliflower with Cheese and Garlic

Ingredients
Servings 4

- 2 Cups of crumbled feta cheese
- 1 medium head of cauliflower
- 2 tablespoons of olive oil
- 2 crushed garlic cloves
- Pepper and salt to taste

Cooking Directions

- Preheat your oven to 400 F.
- Wash your cauliflower head and separate it into small florets.
- Pour cauliflower in a baking pan.
- Add pepper salt and crushed garlic.
- Drizzle 1/4 cup of olive oil over it.
- Bake in the oven for 40 minutes.
- Remove from oven and serve topped with crumbled feta cheese.

Greek Peas-Arakas Latheros

Ingredients
Servings 4

- 2 carrots (sliced)
- 1 lbs. frozen peas
- ½ cup of olive oil
- 1 large potato (cut into bite-size pieces)
- 2 medium tomatoes (grated)
- 1 onion (diced)
- 3 tablespoons of dill (chopped)
- Salt and pepper to taste.

Cooking Directions

- Place a medium-sized pot over heat.
- Add olive oil and sauté onions until soft
- Add potatoes and carrots and sauté for 5 minutes more.
- Add your peas and stir until all the peas are covered in olive oil.
- Add the herbs and spices.
- Stir and bring to a boil.
- Reduce heat and simmer for 30 minutes. Make sure the water has completely evaporated leaving just the olive oil.
- Serve.

Tuscan Tomato and Bread Salad

Ingredients
Servings 4

- 1 tablespoon of olive oil
- 4 slices of stale bread
- 1 large tomato (chopped into bite-size pieces)
- 2 tablespoons of red wine vinegar
- 1 small cucumber (sliced)
- 1 handful of basil (chopped)
- Salt and pepper to taste
- 1 small onion (sliced thinly)

Cooking Directions

- Pour the red wine vinegar into a bowl and add the sliced onions to soak in the vinegar. Set aside.
- In another large bowl, add 4 parts of water to 1 part of vinegar, and add the bread to soak for a few minutes.
- Remove the bread into a colander and press out the liquid.
- Transfer bread into a large salad bowl.
- Add cucumber, tomato, basil, and soaked onions to the bowl. Mix well.
- Add salt, pepper and olive oil. Mix well.
- Place in the refrigerator for an hour.
- Serve drizzled with olive oil.

Greek Marinated Anchovies

Ingredients
Servings 4

- Olive oil (sufficient to cover the fish)
- Red wine vinegar (sufficient to cover the fish)
- 1 lbs. of fresh anchovies
- Parsley
- Peppercorns
- 1 garlic cloves
- 3 tablespoons of kosher salt

Cooking Directions

- Clean your fish and place them in a dish in layers.
- Sprinkle salt on each layer and cover the dish with plastic wrap. Put it in your refrigerator for 6 hours.
- Remove the dish from your refrigerator and wash the fish again before replacing it in the dish the same way it was at first.
- Pour the red wine vinegar and olive oil over the fish, just enough to cover the fish.
- Place it in your refrigerator and let it sit for 5 hours.
- Remove from your refrigerator and rinse well again. Pat dry with paper towel.
- Put the anchovies in an airtight container and add black peppercorns.
- Add enough olive oil to cover the fish and refrigerate.
- Serve sprinkled with parsley or any other herbs of your choice.

Pan-roasted Herbs and Garlic Crusted Sardines

Ingredients
Servings 4

- 2 teaspoons of French mustard
- 1 lbs. of fresh sardines
- 1 tablespoon of lemon juice
- 2 teaspoons of fresh parsley (chopped)
- 1 tablespoon of dried oregano
- Freshly ground pepper to taste
- ¼ teaspoons of salt
- 1 teaspoon dried onion flakes
- ½ teaspoon of paprika
- 1 garlic cloves (minced)

Cooking Directions

- Rinse and pat your sardines dry.
- Preheat your oven to 430 F. Put the oven fan on.
- Combine all the ingredients except parsley and sardines in a large bowl and mix together.
- Add the sardines and toss gently so the herbs coat the fish evenly.
- Place a pan over medium heat and add some olive oil to heat up.
- Put the sardines in the pan and make sure they are all in one layer.
- Roast in the pan for 15 minutes.
- Remove and serve sprinkled with fresh parsley.

Baked Phyllo Chips

Ingredients
Servings 2

- 4 Phyllo sheets
- 1 cup of grated cheese
- Olive oil
- 1 tablespoon of herbs de Provence

Cooking Directions

- Preheat your oven to 350F.
- Spread one Phyllo sheet on a flat work surface and brush it with olive oil.
- Sprinkle herbs and cheese on it.
- Cover it up with a second Phyllo sheet.
- Repeat until you've exhausted all your Phyllo sheets.
- Use a pizza cutter to cut it into small pieces.
- Place each piece in a baking plan lined with parchment paper.
- Place in the oven and bake for 8 minutes.
- Serve or store in an airtight container.

Mediterranean Chicken Orzo

Ingredients
Servings 4

- ¼ cup of pine nuts
- 2 tablespoons of olive oil
- ¼ teaspoon of red pepper flakes
- ¼ cup of white wine
- 1 lb. Chicken breasts (sliced thin and pounded)
- ½ cup of feta
- 1 ½ cup of whole wheat orzo (dried)
- ½ teaspoon of oregano
- 1 ½ cup of grape tomatoes (halved)
- ½ teaspoon of pepper
- ½ tablespoon of minced garlic
- 1 tablespoon of fresh parsley (chopped)
- 1 tablespoon of fresh basil (chopped)
- ½ cup of kalamata olives (pitted and sliced)
- 1 cup of spinach (chopped)

Cooking Directions

- Place a small saucepan over heat and add water. Bring to a boil.
- Add orzo to boiling water and cook according to instructions on the packet. Remove from heat and set aside.
- Place another pan over medium heat and add a tablespoon of olive oil to heat up.
- Cook chicken in the heated oil. Cook for 5 minutes or until all sides turn golden brown.
- Remove chicken from pan and set aside.
- Add another tablespoon of olive oil to the pan.
- Add garlic to the pan and stir-fry for 1 minute.
- Add white wine and cherry tomatoes. Stir.
- Increase the heat to high and let it simmer for 5 minutes.
- Add the cooked orzo, kalamata olives, spices, spinach, and pine nuts. Continue to toss until everything is well combined.

- Serve orzo topped with chickens.

One Pan Healthy Paella

Ingredients
Servings 4

- 1 teaspoon of black pepper
- 1.5 lbs. Boneless chicken breasts (cut into cubes)
- 1 cup of frozen peas
- 2 tablespoons of olive oil (divided into two)
- 3 cups of chicken broth
- ¼ teaspoon of saffron threads
- ½ cup of onion (diced)
- 1 cup of brown rice
- 1 tablespoon of garlic(minced)
- ½ tablespoon of thyme leaves
- 1 ½ cup of thinly sliced bell peppers
- 3 bay leaves
- 2 cups of sugar snap peas
- 1 tablespoon of paprika
- 1 teaspoon of black pepper
- ½ teaspoon of salt
- 1 cup of frozen peas
- 1 tablespoon of lemon juice
- 3 cups of chicken broth

Cooking Directions

- Place a large pan over heat and add a tablespoon of olive oil to heat up.
- Add chicken to the pan and cook for 15 minutes or until all sides turn brown.
- Remove browned chicken from pan and set aside.
- Add another tablespoon of olive oil to the pan. Add garlic and onions; sauté until translucent.
- Add sugar snap peas and peppers. Sauté for 6 minutes or until tender.
- Add dry brown rice and turn up the heat to high. Cook for 5 minutes.

- Add the chicken back into the pan and add spices and chicken stock. Stir everything together. Bring to a boil.
- Reduce heat to low and allow simmer for 30 minutes.
- Add frozen peas and stir.
- Serve.

Greek Chicken Zucchini Noodles

Ingredients
Servings 2

- ½ teaspoon of pepper
- 1 tablespoon of olive oil
- ½ teaspoon of oregano
- 1/3 cup of kalamata olives (halved)
- 3 medium zucchini (spiralized)
- 1 lbs. chicken breasts (cut into ½ inch cubes)
- 1 tablespoon of freshly squeezed lemon juice
- 1 cup of marinated artichoke hearts
- ½ teaspoon of dried oregano
- 1/3 cup of sun-dried tomatoes in olive oil (drained)
- ½ teaspoon dried basil
- ½ teaspoon of thyme

Cooking Directions

- Place a pan over heat and add olive oil to heat up.
- Sauté chicken in the pan for 15 minutes, or until all sides turn completely brown.
- Add spices, artichoke hearts, sun dried tomatoes and olives. Stir and cook for another 3 minutes.
- Add spiralized zucchini and lemon juice and toss. Cook for 2 minutes.
- Serve.

Beef Stuffed Acorn Squash

Ingredients
Servings 4

- 1 lb. ground beef
- 1 cup of cheddar cheese (shredded)
- 2 acorn squash (halved)
- ½ cup of pecans (chopped)
- 1 tablespoon of Walnut oil
- ½ teaspoon of salt
- ½ cup of onion (diced finely)
- 1 teaspoon of pepper
- ½ tablespoon of minced garlic
- 1 teaspoon of fresh sage (chopped)
- 1 lb. ground beef
- 1 teaspoon of rosemary (chopped)
- 1 ½ cups of baby bella mushrooms (chopped)
- ½ cup of chicken stock
- ¼ cup of dried figs (chopped)

Cooking Directions

- Line a baking sheet with parchment paper.
- Preheat your oven to 450F.
- Grease baking sheet with walnut oil.
- Scoop out seeds from the acorn squash and place flat on the baking sheet.
- Bake for 22 minutes or until tender.
- While squash is baking, add a tablespoon of walnut oil to a saucepan placed over low heat.
- Add onions and garlic. Sauté for 3 minutes.
- Add ground beef to the pan and sauté for 10 minutes.
- Add dried figs, herbs, chopped mushrooms, chicken stock, pepper, salt and pecans. Sauté for another 5 minutes.
- Remove baked squash from the oven and scoop out the center, leaving the squash 'boat'.

- Add the scooped out filling to the pan along with your beef and mushrooms mixture. Stir and cook for 2 minutes.
- Now, fill up the boats with the beef filling in the pan and top with cheese.
- Preheat your oven to 450F.
- Place filled squash boats on a greased baking pan and bake in the oven for 10 minutes.
- Serve.

Healthy Baked Ziti

Ingredients
Servings 8

- 1 teaspoon of pepper
- 1 lbs. whole wheat ziti
- 1 teaspoon of garlic powder
- 2 tablespoons of olive oil
- 1 teaspoon of garlic powder
- 1 lbs. ground turkey
- 2 tablespoons of chopped basil
- 14 ounces canned chopped tomatoes
- ¼ cup of parmesan cheese
- 1 cup of ricotta cheese
- 2 cups of mozzarella cheese (divided into two)
- 14 ounces canned tomato sauce

Cooking Directions

- Pre-heat your oven to 350F.
- Grease a 9 by 13 inch baking dish and set aside.
- Place a pot over heat and add water. Bring to a boil.
- Cook ziti in the boiling water for 6 minutes or according to the instructions on the package. Drain and set aside.
- Place another pan over heat and add olive oil to heat up.
- Brown turkey in the pan for 10 minutes or until all sides turns completely brown.
- Add ricotta, parmesan and a cup of mozzarella cheese to a mixing bowl. Add pepper and basil. Mix everything together.
- Add cooked ziti to the cheese mixture and stir.
- Add spices, ground turkey to the cheese mixture and stir.
- Pour the mixture into your prepared baking dish.
- Sprinkle the rest of your mozzarella cheese on top.
- Place in the oven and cook for 30 minutes.
- Serve.

Mediterranean Bento Bowl

Ingredients
Servings 1

- 2 tablespoons of hummus
- 1 tablespoon of parsley (chopped)
- ½ cup of chickpeas (rinsed)
- 1 whole-wheat pita bread (quartered)
- ¼ cup of cucumber (diced)
- 1 cup of grapes
- ¼ cup of tomato (diced)
- 3 ounces turkey breast (grilled)
- 1 tablespoon of olives (diced)
- 1 teaspoon of red wine vinegar
- 1 tablespoon of feta cheese (crumbled)
- ½ teaspoon of extra virgin olive oil

Cooking Directions

- Add cucumber, chickpeas, parsley, tomato, olives, feta, olive oil, and vinegar to a salad bowl and toss to combine.
- Pour the mixture into a medium-sized bowl or lunch box with multiple compartments.
- Heat the grilled turkey in your microwave and place inside another compartment in the lunch box.
- Pack pita and grapes in a separate compartment.
- Add hummus to a separate dip-size container.
- Your bento lunch box is ready to go.

DINNER RECIPES

Moussaka

Ingredients
Servings 2

- 1 tablespoon of olive oil
- ⅔ cup (100g pack)of crumbled feta cheese
- ½ onion (finely chopped)
- 1 cup (200g) can of chickpeas
- 1 garlic clove (finely chopped)
- 1 cup (200g) can of chickpeas
- 9 oz. (250g)lean beef mince
- 1 teaspoon of ground cinnamon
- 1 cup (200g)can of chopped tomatoes
- 1 tablespoon of tomato purée
- For serving: Brown bread

Cooking Directions

- Place a pan over heat and add oil to heat up.
- Add garlic and onion and saute until soft.
- Add mince and stir-fry for 4 minutes.
- Tip tomatoes into the pan. Add tomato puree and stir.
- Add seasoning and cinnamon. Stir.
- Leave to simmer for 10 minutes.
- Add chickpeas and let everything simmer for 10 more minutes.
- Turn off heat and sprinkle with dried mint and feta cheese.
- Serve with toasted bread.

Spiced Tomato Baked Eggs

Ingredients
Servings 2

- 1 tablespoon of olive oil
- 4 eggs
- 4 cups (800g) can of cherry tomatoes
- 2 red onions (chopped)
- One small bunch of coriander stalks
- 1 red chili (deseeded & chopped)
- 1 garlic clove (sliced)
- For serving: Brown bread

Cooking Directions

- Place a frying pan over heat and add oil to heat up.
- Add garlic, chili, coriander stalks, and onions and cook for 5 minutes.
- Add tomatoes, stir and cook for 10 minutes.
- Use the back of a spoon to make 4 holes inside the sauce and crack the eggs in the hole.
- Place a lid on the pan and let it cook over low heat for 7 minutes.
- Top with coriander leaves.
- Serve on top of bread.

Salmon with Potato and Corn Salad

Ingredients
Servings 2

- One handful of basil leaves
- 1 ⅓ cups (200g) of baby new potatoes
- 1 tablespoon of capers (finely chopped)
- 1 sweet corn cob
- One bunch of spring onions/scallions (finely chopped)
- 2 skinless salmon fillets
- 1 tablespoon of extra-virgin olive oil
- ⅓ (60g) cup of tomatoes
- 1 tablespoon of red wine vinegar

Cooking Directions

- Add potatoes to a pot of boiling water and let it cook until tender.
- Combine capers, vinegar, basil, oil, seasoning and spring onions or scallions together.
- Heat up your grill to high heat.
- Rub dressing over salmon.
- Place salmon over the grill with the skin side facing down. Grill for 8 minutes.
- Slice tomatoes and share amongst serving dishes.
- Slice potatoes and share amongst serving dishes.
- Add grilled salmon to serving dishes.
- Drizzle remaining dressing over it.
- Enjoy.

Spiced Carrot and Lentil Soup

Ingredients
Servings 2

- A pinch of chili flakes
- ¼ (60ml) cup of milk
- 1 teaspoon of cumin seeds
- 2 ¼ cups (500ml) of hot vegetable stock
- 1 tablespoon of olive oil
- ⅓ cup (70g) of split red lentils
- 2 cups (300g) of carrots (washed and coarsely grated)
- For serving: Greek yogurt

Cooking Directions

- Place a large saucepan over heat and chili flakes and season flakes. Dryfry for 1 minute.
- Scoop out half of the cumin and pepper mixture and set aside.
- Add oil to the remaining seed and add stock, lentils, carrots and milk. Bring to a boil.
- Let it simmer for 15 minutes.
- Scoop the soup into a blender or food processor and puree until smooth.

Mediterranean Chicken Quinoa & Greek Salad

Ingredients
Servings 2

- ½ cup (50g) of crumbled feta cheese
- ⅗ (100g) cup of quinoa
- Juice and zest of ½ lemon
- ½ red chili (deseeded and finely chopped)
- One small bunch of mint leaves (chopped)
- 1 garlic clove (crushed)
- 2 chicken breasts
- ½ red onion (finely sliced)
- 1 tablespoon of extra-virgin olive oil
- One handful of pitted black kalamata olives
- ¾ cup (150g) of tomatoes (roughly chopped)

Cooking Directions

- Cook Quinoa according to the instructions on the package.
- Drain quinoa and set aside.
- Toss chicken fillets in olive oil and sprinkle seasoning, olive oil, garlic, and salt over it.
- Place the chicken fillets in a heated pan to cook for 4 minutes.
- Flip fillets and cook for another 3 minutes.
- Remove and set aside.
- Combine olives, feta cheese, tomatoes, mint and onions in a bowl and toss.
- Add quinoa and toss.
- Stir through the remaining olive oil, zest, lemon juice and seasoning.
- Serve with chicken on top.

Grilled Vegetables with Bean Mash

Ingredients
Servings 2

- 1 tablespoon of chopped coriander
- 1 pepper (deseeded & quartered)
- ½ (100ml) cup vegetable stock
- 1 aubergine (sliced lengthways)
- 1 garlic clove (crushed)
- 2 courgettes (sliced lengthways)
- 2 cups (400g can) of haricot beans (rinsed)
- 2 tablespoons of olive oil

Cooking Directions

- Heat up your grill.
- Arrange your veggies in a grill pan and brush lightly with olive oil.
- Place on grill, and grill until the veggies turn light brown.
- Flip veggies over and brush again with olive oil.
- Grill until tender.
- While the veggies are roasting, place a pan over heat and add beans, stock and garlic. Bring to a boil.
- Let it simmer for 10 minutes.
- Use a potato masher to mash roughly.
- Divide roasted veggies amongst serving plates.
- Divide mash amongst serving plates.
- Drizzle oil over the dishes.
- Sprinkle with coriander and black pepper.
- Serve.

Spicy Mediterranean Beet Salad

Ingredients
Servings 2

- 8 raw baby beetroots (scrubbed)
- 1 teaspoon of crushed red chili flakes
- ½ tablespoon of sumac
- 1 tablespoon of Harissa paste
- ½ tablespoon of ground cumin
- ½ (200g) cup of Greek yogurt
- 2 cups (400g) can chickpeas (drained and rinsed)
- ½ teaspoon of lemon juice
- 2 tablespoons of olive oil
- ½ teaspoon of lemon zest
- For serving: mint leaves (chopped)

Cooking Directions

- Heat up your oven to 425F/220C.
- Quarter your beetroots.
- Combine all your spices together.
- Place beetroots and chickpeas on a large baking tray and season with spices.
- Add pepper and salt to taste.
- Place in the oven and roast for 30 minutes.
- Meanwhile, combine lemon juice with lemon zest and yogurt.
- Swirl harrisa through and spread in a bowl.
- Remove chickpeas and beetroot.
- Sprinkle with mint leaves and crushed red flakes.
- Serve.

Honey Lemon Chicken Laps

Ingredients
Servings 4

- 3 garlic cloves (slice each clove in half)
- 7 chicken laps
- 1 ½ tablespoons of honey
- 1 tablespoon of olive oil
- Salt and pepper to taste
- 2 tablespoons of lemon juice

Cooking Directions

- Preheat your oven to 400F.
- Wash and pat chicken laps dry with a paper towel.
- Sprinkle salt and pepper over chickens and set aside to marinate for a few minutes.
- Place a medium-sized oven-safe pan over heat and add olive oil and lemon juice. Let it heat up.
- Now, add a sprinkle of pepper and your honey. Stir and let the honey heat up.
- Scoop some of the honey-lemon mixture from the pan.
- Put all your chicken laps in the pan making sure the laps are in one layer.
- Now, drizzle the honey lemon mixture you scooped out earlier over the chicken laps.
- Put one garlic halve on top of each chicken lap.
- Remove pan from heat and place in the oven.
- Bake for 30 minutes.
- Use a prong to remove the chicken laps to your serving dishes.
- Serve with leftover honey lemon mixture served over the chicken laps as sauce.

Grilled Chicken Skewers served with Vegetable Salad

Ingredients
Servings 4

- 1 lbs. chicken breasts (Cut into 1 inch cubes)
- Juice of 1 lemon
- 1 teaspoon of dried oregano
- ¼ cup of extra virgin olive oil
- ½ teaspoon of salt
- 3 cloves of garlic (minced)

Cooking Directions

- Combine lemon juice, olive oil, salt, garlic, dried oregano in a bowl and whisk well.
- Pour the mixture in a Ziploc bag and add chicken breast cubes. Shake well and put the bag in your refrigerator for 1-2 hours.
- Remove chicken from Ziploc bag and skewer.
- Grill on medium heat for 15 minutes, flip and grill the other side for 10 minutes.
- Serve with vegetable salad of choice.

Cod and Asparagus Bake

Ingredients
Servings 4

- 1 pint of cherry tomatoes (halved)
- ¼ cup of Romano cheese (grated)
- 4 pieces of 4-ounce Cod fillets
- 2 tablespoons of lemon juice and 1s½ teaspoons of grated lemon zest
- 1 lbs. fresh thin asparagus (trimmed)

Cooking Directions

- Preheat your oven to 375F.
- Put your cod and asparagus in a baking dish.
- Arrange tomatoes on the sides with the skin side facing up.
- Sprinkle all other ingredients inside the dish.
- Bake in your oven for 12 minutes.
- While it is baking, preheat your broiler.
- Broil for 3 minutes.
- Serve.

Lemon Chicken with Asparagus

Ingredients
Servings 4

- 2 cups of asparagus (chopped)
- 2 tablespoons of butter
- 2 tablespoons of honey
- ¼ cup of flour
- 1 teaspoon of lemon pepper seasoning and salt to taste
- 1 lbs. boneless, skinless chicken breasts

Cooking Directions

- Cut chicken breasts in half horizontally to get ¾ inch thick slices.
- Pour flour in a shallow dish and add salt and pepper. Mix.
- Add chicken breast slices to the dish and toss so the flour mix coats the chicken.
- Place a medium-sized skillet over heat and add 2 tablespoons of butter to melt.
- Add the honey and stir.
- Add chicken and stir. Sauté for about 5 minutes or until all sides are browned.
- Sprinkle lemon pepper over cooked chicken. Stir and remove chickens from the pan.
- Add asparagus to the pan and sauté until tender and crisp. Serve with chickens.
- Serve with lemon wedges on the side.

Sweet and Easy Herb- baked Sweet Potatoes

Ingredients
Servings 4

- 4 medium-sized sweet potatoes (rinsed, scrubbed and cut in half lengthwise)
- ½ teaspoon each of coriander, cinnamon, cumin, and paprika mixed together
- 1 15-ounce can of chickpeas (rinsed and drained)
- Sea salt and lemon juice to taste
- ½ tablespoon of olive oil

Cooking Directions

- Preheat your oven to 400F.
- Line a large-sized baking dish with parchment paper.
- Pour chickpeas in your prepared baking dish and drizzle spices and olive oil over it. Toss.
- Rub olive oil over the potatoes and sprinkle the herbs mixture over it.
- Place herb coated potatoes in the baking dish alongside the chickpeas.
- Roast in the oven for 45 minutes.
- Serve.

Cauliflower Rice with Rotini Pasta and Sausage

Ingredients
Servings 4

- 5 tablespoons of olive oil
- 12 ounces rotini pasta (Cook with ½ cup of water)
- 5 cups of cauliflower rice
- 1 teaspoon of lemon zest
- ¾ lbs. sweet Italian bulk sausage
- 1 teaspoon of dried oregano
- ½ cup of chopped fresh flat-leaf parsley
- 1 teaspoon of garlic powder

Cooking Directions

- Place a skillet over medium heat and add a tablespoon of olive oil.
- Use a spoon to break up the sausage and add it to the skillet. Brown the sausage in the skillet for 6 minutes.
- Removed browned sausage to a bowl.
- Add cooed cauliflower rice to the skillet along with garlic powder and oregano. Stir.
- Add the remaining olive oil to the pan and stir.
- Add in all other ingredients and stir.
- Serve.

Classic Greek Lemon Roasted Chicken and Potatoes

Ingredients
Servings 4

- 2 tablespoons of lemon juice
- 1.5 lbs. chicken thighs
- 3 allspice berries
- 2 lbs. potatoes (Cut each potato into half wedges)
- ¾ cup of olive oil
- 2 tablespoons of dried oregano
- 2 garlic cloves
- 3 cloves
- ½ teaspoon of salt
- Pepper to taste

Cooking Directions

- Preheat your oven 375 F.
- Wash and pat your chicken thighs dry. Rub in a pinch of salt, oregano and pepper.
- Brush with olive oil and set aside.
- Put the potato wedges in a bowl and add lemon juice, ½ cup of olive oil, ½ teaspoon of salt, ½ tablespoon of oregano, and some spices.
- Make sure the herbs, spices and oil coat the potatoes all round.
- Pour the potatoes in a baking pan. Make sure it is all in one layer.
- Add the chicken on top of the potatoes.
- Add allspice berries.
- Add garlic cloves and cloves.
- Pour some hot water in one corner of the pan. Don't pour the water over the potatoes so it doesn't rinse off the spices.
- Tilt the pan to one corner so that the water you put in covers the potatoes halfway.
- Place in the oven to roast for 15 minutes.

- Reduce the heat of your oven to 320F and roast for another 45 minutes.
- Serve.

Grilled Honey Harrissa Chicken Skewers served with Garlicky Mint Sauce

Ingredients
Servings 4

- 3 tablespoons of Greek yoghurt
- 6 tablespoons of olive oil
- 2 chicken breasts (skinless, boneless and cut into ½ inch strips)
- 3 tablespoons of mild harrisa
- 1 tablespoon of honey
- 1 tablespoon of fresh mint (chopped)
- ½ teaspoon of salt
- ¼ teaspoon of freshly ground black pepper
- 3 garlic cloves
- 3 tablespoons of lemon juice

Cooking Directions

- Combine 1 tablespoon of olive oil, harrissa, honey, ¼ teaspoon of ground pepper and ½ teaspoon of salt in a bowl and mix.
- Add chicken and mix well.
- Cover the bowl and place in your refrigerator for 1 hour to marinate.
- Soak wooden skewers in water for 30 minutes.
- Arrange chicken strips on skewers horizontally.
- Grill for 4 minutes on each side.
- Add 3 garlic cloves (crushed), 1 tablespoon of chopped mint, 5 tablespoons of olive oil, 3 tablespoons of yoghurt, 3 tablespoons of lemon juice to your food processor and process until smooth.
- Serve sauce over honey harrissa chicken skewers.

Greek-inspired Baked Mac and Cheese

Ingredients
Servings 4

- ½ Cup of Greek yoghurt
- ½ pound of pasta
- 1/4 cups of olives (chopped)
- 3 ounces of feta cheese and 3 tablespoons of cream cheese
- 1 tablespoon of olive oil
- 1 tablespoon of parsley
- 1 tablespoon of mint
- 1 tablespoon of dried oregano
- Salt and pepper to taste
- 1 chopped onion
- 1 chopped pepper

Cooking Directions

- Preheat your oven to 350 F.
- Cook your pasta according to the instructions on the package.
- Place a saucepan over medium heat.
- Add 1 1/2 tablespoon of olive oil to the pan. Let the oil heat up.
- Add chopped onions and pepper sauté until softened.
- Add the olives and all your herbs. Sauté for 2 minutes.
- Mash the feta cheese in a bowl, and add cream cheese and yoghurt. Mix together until creamy, and then add some pepper.
- Add the cooked and drained pasta to the pot with the herbs and veggies. Mix well.
- Add the remaining olive oil and mix well.
- Add your cheese sauce and mix well.
- Pour everything in a casserole dish and bake it in the oven for 20 minutes.
- Serve.

Greek-styled Juicy Roasted Meatballs

Ingredients
Servings 4

- ¼ cup of olive oil
- 2 tablespoons of red wine vinegar
- 1 Pound of ground beef
- 2 tablespoons of breadcrumbs
- All-purpose flour
- ⅓ cup of fresh mint (chopped)
- ½ teaspoon of sea salt
- Pepper to taste
- ½ teaspoon of cumin
- 1 tablespoon of orzo.

Cooking Directions

- Preheat your oven to 350F.
- Pour beef in a large bowl and add 2 tablespoons of olive oil.
- Add the remaining ingredients except all-purpose flour and olive oil.
- Mix the beef and the other ingredients together until well incorporated.
- Roll into 1 1/2 inch thick meatballs.
- Use some olive oil to brush a baking pan lightly.
- Arrange the meatballs in the baking pan and brush each ball lightly with olive oil.
- Bake for 15 minutes, flip halfway and bake for another 15 minutes.
- Broil for 5 minutes.
- Serve.

Stewed Pork and Greens in Lemon Sauce

Ingredients
Servings 4

- 4 allspice berries
- Juice from 2 lemons
- 2 lbs. of pork shoulder (cut into large chunks)
- 2 lbs. of Swiss chard (roughly chopped)
- 1 white leek (sliced)
- ½ cup of olive oil
- ½ cup of dill (chopped)
- 2 bay leaves
- 4 spring onions (sliced)
- 4 onions (chopped)

Cooking Directions

- Place a heavy pan over medium heat and add two spoons of olive oil to heat up.
- Add all the herbs and spices then add the meat. Brown the meat for 3 minutes on each side.
- Place another pot over heat and add your remaining olive oil.
- Add onions and sauté for 2 minutes.
- Add spring onions and leek. Sauté until soft.
- Add dill and sauté for another 1 minute.
- Add your ground meat and salt and pepper to taste add some water to cover the meat cover the pot and cook for 1 hour until the meat is tender.
- Add lemon juice and chard to the pot.
- Stir well and allow simmer for 20 minutes.
- Serve.

Greek Chicken Cooked in Diced Tomato

Ingredients
Servings 3

- 2 onions (diced)
- 4 Allspice berries
- 20 ounces fresh tomatoes (diced)
- 1.5 lbs. Chicken breasts (cut into pieces)
- 2 ½ tablespoons of olive oil
- 1 teaspoon of salt
- 2 garlic cloves (minced)
- 1 bay leaf
- 1 cinnamon sticks
- Pepper to taste

Cooking Directions

- Place a large deep pan over medium heat and add olive oil to heat up.
- Add your chicken pieces and brown both sides for 10 minutes.
- Use a spoon to push the browned chicken pieces aside and add onions to the pan. Sauté until soft.
- Add garlic and sauté for 1 minute.
- Add all other ingredients and add 1/3 cup of water. Stir and allow simmer for 45 minutes.
- Serve over rice or pasta.

Roasted Veggies Pita Pizza

Ingredients
Servings 6

- 6 whole wheat mini pita breads
- 3 tablespoons of tomato paste and 1 cup of cherry tomatoes (halved)
- 1 eggplant (sliced thinly)
- 4 tablespoons of olive oil
- 1 zucchini (sliced thinly)
- Feta cheese
- 1 tablespoon of dried oregano
- 1 clove of garlic (sliced thinly)
- 1 onion (sliced thinly)

Cooking Directions

- Preheat the oven to 400 F
- Combine your eggplant, garlic, zucchini, and onions in a bowl.
- Add a pinch of salt and 3 tablespoons of olive oil and mix.
- Add oregano and use your hands to mix it very well.
- Add your tomato halves to a bowl and mix with one teaspoon of olive oil.
- Pour the zucchini mixture into a pan and push it to the side
- Add tomatoes to the side of the zucchini.
- Place it in the oven to roast for 20 minutes.
- While the veggies are roasting, make your tomato sauce by combining the tomato paste with olive oil and 4 tablespoons of water.
- Add some oregano and stir until you get a thick consistency
- Place pita bread in the bottom of a pan and spread the tomato sauce on top of the pita bread.
- Top with zucchini mixture and roasted tomatoes
- Drizzle 1/4 teaspoon of olive oil on the pita bread.
- Place in the oven to bake for 15 minutes.
- Serve topped with crumbled feta cheese.

Italian Sheet Pan Eggs with Prosciutto and Artichokes

Ingredients
Servings 2

- 5 eggs
- 4 slices of prosciutto
- 1 tablespoon of olive oil
- 5 cherry tomatoes (quartered)
- 3 canned artichoke hearts (roughly diced)
- ¼ teaspoon of pepper
- ½ teaspoon of sea salt
- 1 tablespoon of fresh oregano leaves (chopped)
- 1 scallion (diced)

Cooking Directions

- Preheat your oven to 355F.
- Brush a sheet pan with olive oil.
- Crack eggs into the pan.
- Scatter all other ingredients except prosciutto over it.
- Place the pan in the oven and bake for 8 minutes until the egg white is set.
- Remove from oven and sprinkle prosciutto over it.
- Serve.

Israeli Yellow Chicken and Potatoes

Ingredients
Servings 4

- 4 chicken legs quarters (sliced)
- 2 pounds of potatoes (cut into long strips)
- 2 tablespoons of olive oil
- 1 large onion (sliced)
- Salt and pepper to taste
- 3 teaspoons of turmeric
- 2 teaspoons of chicken bouillon powder

Cooking Directions

- Wash chickens and pat dry.
- Place a pan over heat and add the oil to heat up.
- Add chickens to the pan and fry until all sides turn golden brown.
- Remove chickens and add onions to the pan. Sauté until slightly browned.
- Add potatoes and fry until golden brown on all sides.
- Add chickens back in the pan and sprinkle bouillon powder and turmeric over it.
- Add 2 cup of water. Bring to boil.
- Reduce heat to low and continue to cook until potatoes are softened.
- Sprinkle salt and pepper.
- Serve.

Israeli Green Rice

Ingredients
Servings 6

- 1 ½ cups of Basmati rice
- Extra virgin olive oil
- 3 garlic cloves (minced)
- 2 shallots (sliced thinly)
- Kosher salt
- Freshly ground black pepper to taste
- 2 cups of mixed and chopped herbs(tarragon, dill, mint, parsley, basil)

Cooking Directions

- Pour 3 cups of water in a pot and bring to a boil.
- Place a skillet over medium heat and add a small quantity of olive oil to heat up.
- Add shallots and sauté until golden brown.
- Add garlic and sauté for 1 minute more.
- Add the rice and continue to stir until the rice turns opaque.
- Now, add the boiling water and cover the pan while the rice continues to simmer for 15 minutes.
- Turn off the heat but don't open the pot. Let it sit for 10 minutes so the steam can finish the cooking.
- Add your chopped herbs and stir.
- Serve.

Italian Hot Dish Dinner

Ingredients
Servings 4

- 1 ½ cups of multigrain bow tie pasta
- ½ cup of shredded mozzarella cheese (part-skim)
- 2 tablespoons of grated parmesan cheese
- 1 15 ounce can of tomato sauce
- 1 lbs. lean ground beef
- 1 cup of fresh mushrooms (sliced)
- 1/8 teaspoon of pepper
- 1 teaspoon of dried oregano
- ¼ teaspoon of onion powder
- ½ teaspoon of garlic powder
- ½ cup of chopped green pepper
- ½ cup of chopped onions

Cooking Directions

- Preheat your oven to 350F.
- Cook pasta according to the instructions on the package. Drain and set aside.
- Place a large skillet over medium heat and spray it with cooking spray.
- Add the beef to the skillet along with the chopped green onions, chopped peppers and mushrooms. Cook for 7 minutes.
- Add tomato sauce and seasonings. Stir and bring to a boil.
- Allow simmer for 15 minutes.
- Turn off the heat.
- Spray an 8 inch baking dish with cooking spray and add your cooked pasta to it.
- Sprinkle a tablespoon of parmesan cheese and ¼ cup of mozzarella cheese on it.
- Place in the oven to bake for 35 minutes.
- Remove from oven and sprinkle the remaining cheese on it.
- Return to the oven and bake for another 7 minutes.
- Serve with sauce.

Easy Pasta Skillet Dinner

Ingredients
Servings 8

- 1 8 ounce can of tomato sauce
- 1 lbs. Italian turkey sausage (remove casings)
- 1 6 ounce pack of baby spinach leaves
- 1 8 ounce can of salt-free tomato sauce
- 3 ½ cups of dry multigrain farfalle pasta
- ½ cup of mozzarella cheese (shredded)
- 1 14 ounce can of diced tomatoes
- Basil, garlic and oregano

Cooking Directions

- Spray a large sized skillet with cooking spray.
- Place the skillet over medium heat.
- Add sausage to the skillet and crumble. Stir-cook until it loses its pink color.
- Pour the can of diced tomatoes with the herbs in without draining the juice. Stir.
- Add tomato sauce, pasta, and 1 ¼ cups of water. Stir.
- Bring to a boil.
- Cook for 15 minutes.
- Add spinach and stir.
- Cook until spinach wilts.
- Serve with cheese sprinkled over it.

Easy Minestrone Soup Dinner

Ingredients
Servings 4

- 2 tablespoons of grape seed oil
- 2 carrots (peeled and diced)
- 1 796 ML can of diced organic tomatoes
- ¾ cup of any gluten-free pasta
- 1 540 ML can of red kidney beans
- 2 cups of chopped kale
- ¼ cup of chopped fresh basil
- ¼ teaspoon of chili flakes
- 1 minced garlic clove
- 1 diced celery stalk
- 1 diced onion

Cooking Directions

- Place a large pot over medium heat.
- Add grape seed oil to heat up then add your carrots, onions, garlic and celery. Cook for 3 minutes.
- Add pasta, beans, tomatoes, chili flakes, and a cup of boiling water. Bring to a boil.
- Cook for 11 minutes.
- Add the chopped kale and turn off the heat.
- Serve sprinkled with fresh basil.

Healthy Lasagna

Ingredients
Servings 8

- ½ lbs. ground beef
- 2 medium-sized zucchini (Cut into ½ inch cubes)
- 15 ounce can of whole tomatoes with a 10 ounce can of tomato sauce
- 1 medium-sized summer squash (Cut into ½ inch cubes)
- 6 lasagna noodles (uncooked)
- 1 cup of shredded mozzarella cheese
- ½ cup of grated parmesan cheese
- 10-ounce small curd cottage cheese
- Salt and pepper to taste
- 1 teaspoon of dried basil
- ½ teaspoon of dried parsley
- ½ teaspoon of garlic powder
- ¼ onion (chopped)

Cooking Directions

- Preheat your oven to 375F.
- Place a skillet over medium heat and add a teaspoon of oil to heat up.
- Add onions and ground beef. Stir-cook until the beef is fully cooked. Set aside to drain.
- Pour diced zucchini and summer squash into the pan and cook for 10 minutes.
- Add tomatoes, tomato sauce, and all of your herbs and seasonings.
- Cook over medium heat for 15 minutes.
- Add the beef and stir.
- Pour half of the sauce into an 8 by 10 casserole dish.
- Put 3 of the lasagna noodles on top of the sauce.
- Cover it up with half of the tomato sauce you have left.
- Add the half of all your cheese on top.
- Repeat the steps again starting the remaining tomato sauce and then the lasagna noodles and cheese.

- Cover the dish with foil paper and bake in the oven for 15 minutes.
- Serve.

North African Spiced Carrots

Ingredients
Servings 6

- ¼ cup of fresh parsley (chopped)
- 1 tablespoon of extra virgin olive oil
- 1/8 teaspoon of salt
- 4 garlic cloves (minced)
- 3 tablespoons of lemon juice
- 2 teaspoons of paprika
- 1 cup of water
- 1 teaspoon of ground cumin
- 3 cups of sliced carrots
- 1 teaspoon of ground coriander

Cooking Directions

- Place a large nonstick pan over medium heat and add your garlic, coriander, cumin and paprika. Stir-fry for 20 seconds.
- Add lemon juice and carrots. Stir.
- Add salt and stir. Bring to a boil.
- Reduce heat to low, cover the pan and let it cook for another 5 minutes.
- Check that the carrots are tender, then let it cook for 4 minutes or until the liquid turns into a thick syrup.
- Remove from heat and serve.

North African Spiced Shrimps with Couscous

Ingredients
Servings 2

- 1 tablespoon of Ras El Hanout sauce
- 10 ounces of Shrimp
- 2 tablespoons of tomato paste
- 1 cup of couscous
- 1 ounce of pitted dates (roughly chopped)
- 4 cloves of garlic
- ½ bunch of kale (discard the stems and chop roughly)
- 2 scallions (roots chopped off. Separate white bottoms from green tops and slice each part thinly)
- 1 lemon(slice into 2 and deseed)
- 2 teaspoons of lemon zest
- 1 large carrot (peeled and diced)

Cooking Directions

- Place a small pot over heat and a cup of water. Add a pinch of salt and bring to a boil.
- Add couscous and stir. Cover the pot and let it cook for 5 minutes.
- Remove couscous from heat and let it stand for 5 minutes or until the couscous absorbs all of the water.
- Fluff with a fork.
- Place a sauce pan over medium heat and add 2 teaspoons of olive oil to heat up.
- Add the carrots and stir. Season with pepper and salt and continue to stir-fry for 3 minutes.
- Add the white part of the scallions, half of your ras el hanout, and your garlic. Stir-fry for 1 minute.
- Add tomato paste and stir. Cook for 2 minutes.
- Add dates, kale, and a cup of water, pepper and salt to taste. Stir. Cook for 3 minutes while stirring occasionally.
- Add cooked couscous and lemon zest. Cook for 2 minutes.
- Turn off the heat and add juice of half lemon and wedges. Stir.

- Remove from heat and set aside.
- Pat shrimps dry with paper towel.
- Place dried shrimps in a bowl and season with the rest of your Ras el Hanout, pepper and salt.
- Place a pan over heat and add olive oil to heat up.
- Add shrimps to the pan and fry until it turns opaque.
- Reduce heat and add juice of 1 lemon.
- Adjust seasoning.
- Serve couscous with shrimps on top.
- Garnish with the green part of your scallions.

One Pan Mediterranean Chicken

Ingredients
Servings 5

- 1 cup of cherry tomatoes (halved)
- 1 tablespoon of olive oil
- 1 tablespoon of fresh basil
- 1 teaspoon of olive oil
- 1 tablespoon of fresh basil
- 1 ½ pounds lbs. boneless chicken
- 1 tablespoon of fresh oregano
- 1 medium red onion (chopped)
- ½ cup of California ripe black olives (sliced)
- Salt and pepper to taste
- 1 15 ounce can of diced tomatoes

Cooking Directions

- Place a large cast iron skillet over medium heat and add olive oil to heat up.
- Brown your chicken in the skillet for 10 minutes or until all sides are browned.
- Remove browned chicken and set aside.
- Add another tablespoon of oil to the skillet and sauté your onions in the skillet for 2 minutes.
- Add garlic and sauté for 1 minute more.
- Add olives and stir.
- Add canned tomatoes with the juice and cook for 7 minutes.
- Add tomato halves and chickens. Stir. Let it cook for 1 minute.
- Serve with rice or potatoes.

Smoky Tempeh Tostadas with Mango Cabbage Slaw

Ingredients
Servings 3

- ¼ teaspoon of salt
- 1 8-ounce pack of tempeh (cut into thin chunks)
- 1 teaspoon of agave nectar
- ¼ cup of soy sauce
- 1 teaspoon of apple cider vinegar
- 1 teaspoon of chili powder
- 1 tablespoon of fresh lime juice
- 1 teaspoon of hot sauce (or half teaspoon if you don't want it too hot)
- ½ cup of cilantro (finely minced)
- ½ teaspoon of ground cumin
- ¾ cup of mangoes (diced)
- ½ teaspoon of liquid smoke
- 1 ½ cups of red cabbage
- ½ teaspoon of garlic powder
- ¼ teaspoon of black pepper
- 6 corn tortillas
- 1/2 teaspoon of onion powder
- Oil for cooking
- Optional Toppings: Avocado slices, lettuce, cilantro, salsa.

Cooking Directions
- Preheat your oven to 350F.
- Add the tempeh chunks to a bowl.
- In a separate bowl, add the chili powder, liquid smoke, soy sauce, cumin, hot sauce, onions, garlic and chili powder. Whisk everything together.
- Pour the mixture over the tempeh chunks. Toss tempeh chunks so the sauce coats it evenly.
- Add corn tortillas to a baking sheet and brush it lightly with olive oil.

- Bake for 10 minutes until golden and crisp. Set aside and keep warm.
- Place a skillet over heat and add tempeh to the skillet.
- Cook for 5 minutes.
- Combine mango, red cabbage, agave nectar, lime juice, vinegar and salt in a separate bowl and whisk.
- Serve tortillas with tempeh and slaw scooped on top of it.

Sweet Potato Noodles with Almond Sauce

Ingredients
Servings 4

For Sweet Potato Noodles:

- ½ cup of toasted, salted almonds (roughly chopped)
- 2 tablespoons of extra virgin olive oil
- Freshly ground black pepper and salt to taste
- 3 sweet potatoes (spiralized into noodles)
- 4 cups of kale (roughly chopped)

For Almond Sauce:

- 2 tablespoons of Dijon mustard
- 2 tablespoons of extra virgin olive oil
- 2 cups of plain, unsweetened almond milk
- 3 shallots (minced)
- 3 tablespoons of all-purpose flour
- 2 garlic cloves (minced)

Cooking Directions

- Place a medium sized pot over medium heat and add olive oil to heat up.
- Add garlic and shallots; sauté for a minute.
- Add your all-purpose flour and stir continuously for 1 minute.
- Add almond flour and whisk as you add to prevent lumps from forming.
- Let it simmer for 5 minutes.
- Add salt and pepper and stir.
- Add Dijon mustard and whisk for a minute.
- Place the lid on the pot, reduce the heat to low, and let it simmer for 5 minutes.
- Meanwhile, place a large sauce pan over another burner. Add olive oil to heat up.
- Set the heat to medium and add the potato noodles. Sauté for 5 minutes.

- Add kale and cook until it wilts.
- By now, your sauce should be ready, add it to the noodles. Stir so the sauce coats the noodles well.
- Add chopped almonds and toss.
- Season with salt and pepper.
- Serve.

Conclusion

Thank you for purchasing this book. I hope I have been able to provide you with useful information for improving your health and managing your weight.

It is my utmost wish and prayer that after reading this book and using the information you have learned, you will be able to live a healthy and happy life.

If you enjoyed reading this book, please kindly spread the word and tell your friends and family about it or better still, gift them a copy of this book.

Cheers to your good health!

Printed in the USA
CPSIA information can be obtained
at www.ICGtesting.com
LVHW040247271123
765001LV00009B/317